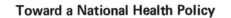

Toward a National Health Policy

Toward a National Health Policy

Public Policy and the Control of Health-Care Costs

Edited by

Kenneth M. Friedman
Purdue University

Stuart H. Rakoff
United Mine Workers of America
Health and Retirement Funds

Lexington Books
D.C. Heath and Company
Lexington, Massachusetts
Toronto

Library of Congress Cataloging in Publication Data
Main entry under title:

Toward a national health policy.

Includes bibliographical references.
1. Medical care—United States—Cost control. 2. Medical care, Cost of—United States. 3. Medical policy—United States. I. Friedman, Kenneth Michael. II. Rakoff, Stuart H.
RA410.53.T68   362.1'0973   75-42931
ISBN 0-669-00563-0

Second printing, June 1978

Published simultaneously in Canada

Printed in the United States of America

International Standard Book Number: 0-669-00563-0

Library of Congress Catalog Card Number: 75-42931

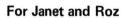

For Janet and Roz

Contents

List of Tables

Acknowledgments

Not too many years ago the number of political scientists interested in the politics of health care could have been counted on one hand. Today, perhaps reflecting the increasing public attention being paid to health issues, a number of political scientists are writing and working in the health area. Much of the credit for this development, and for this book, must go to Professor Ralph Straetz of New York University, who, through his extended guardianship of the Committee on Health Politics, and now his editorship of the *Journal of Health Politics, Policy and Law*, has encouraged and fostered political research into health policy and politics.

The chapters in this volume are revised versions of papers delivered at two panel meetings sponsored by the Committee on Health Politics at the 1975 Annual Meeting of the American Political Science Association in San Francisco. These panels brought together a number of people working on various aspects of the health policy question, both political scientists and others, and established an interaction between authors and other participants that is reflected in the high quality of the analyses that follow. We express our appreciation and respect for the contributors, and trust they have learned as much from each other as we have learned from them collectively.

The opinions and views of the authors are their own, and do not represent those of the organizations with which they are affiliated.

Part I

Introduction

1

Health, Health Costs, and Public Policy

Kenneth M. Friedman
and *Stuart H. Rakoff*

Health-care policy in the United States shows signs of becoming the major domestic issue of the late 1970s and early 1980s. In the context of incremental and often disjointed policy decisions that characterize the American political process, we now seem to have achieved an initial consensus that new public action is required in this area. What is missing, and what may take years to achieve, is the translation of this generalized concern into actionable proposals and workable public programs. Along the way lie a number of obstacles, not the least of which is the necessity to define more clearly the problems that require public action and the activities that will remedy them. The costs and benefits of such proposals must be evaluated to decide if the public desires or can afford proposed programs; at this time remarkably little is known about the costs and benefits of possible public actions.

Three characteristics of the health-care system in the United States provide explanations for both the demands for public action, and the targets of proposed actions. The debate on health policy has taken, and will continue to take, these characteristics as its starting point, and they provide the basis for whatever policies will eventually be enacted:

1. The peculiar undefinable nature of the product, "health"
2. The size, both absolute and relative, and rate of growth of private and public health-care expenditures
3. The disjointed nature of the suppliers of health care, and the essentially oligopsonist (few buyer-many seller) nature of the health-care market.

These characteristics define a system in which traditional methods of public regulation and action may be insufficient to control problems and excesses in the system, a system that has defied rationalization and control. They provide the backdrop against which the chapters in this book must be viewed.

The Nature of the Product – Health as a Commodity

One of the most difficult tasks in dealing with health policy is to define the outputs or outcomes from the health industry. Although it is relatively easy to estimate the inputs in labor, capital, and other costs, the product itself is elusive, and it is difficult to establish a link between inputs and outcomes.

3

Victor Fuchs has commented that "no country is as healthy as it could be; no country does as much for the sick as it is technically capable of doing."[1] In addition, no national consensus has been reached on the objectives of health policy; although better health is the goal, *health* itself is an almost indefinable commodity.

René Dubos has called health "an illusion" and an "undefinable ideal," representing some notion of well-being. He writes in his book *Mirage of Health: Utopias, Progress and Biological Change* that "the illusion that perfect health and happiness are within man's possibilities has flourished in many different forms throughout history."[2] Although it may be illusion and myth, it is clear that governments (our own in particular) strive towards this indefinable ideal. No basic quantifiable minimal health levels or goals have ever been established and accepted and they are impossible to intuit from present or proposed health legislation. Rather, we speak of health care as a right, without specifying at all what we mean. Like the pursuit of happiness, the pursuit of health by government, and by the people, appears to be an inalienable right, which cannot be operationalized in a collective sense, but which (like money) drives and motivates individuals and their political representatives.

Although health itself is difficult to define or measure, health statisticians have become adept at measuring more tangible products of the medical-care industry. We know rather precisely the number of hospital beds filled and vacant, clinic or doctor visits made, and surgical procedures performed. We count the dollars spent on medical care, the pills prescribed, and the diagnostic tests ordered. Centralization of financing of medical care in government and large private third-party payers has improved the reporting of services, and probably has encouraged production of more services at the same time. But increasingly the question is being raised of whether more services or more dollars or more facilities really mean more health.

Many writers and policy leaders have questioned the contribution that increased medical expenditures make to health. Although *per-capita* health-care expenditures are higher in the United States than in any other country there is no clear relationship between these expenditures and health outcomes.[3] Our level of health (as measured by life expectancy and disability) is lower than in other industrialized nations that spend less.[4] Relatively high infant-mortality rates and comparatively unimpressive life-expectancy rates suggest that the marginal utility of additional increases in health-care expenditures may be questionable. These data also suggest the large variance in health status between groups (rich and poor, black and white), differences not amenable to easy manipulation by simply increasing health-care funds. Stephen Strickland has articulated the same point with regard to biomedical research expenditures, where decreasing marginal returns on investment have fostered more specifically directed and goal-oriented research efforts in recent years, such as wars on cancer, heart disease, and sickle cell anemia.[5]

The conceptualization of this problem by Ivan Illich, Rick Carlson, and others in the so-called "end-of-medicine school"[a] appears to be gaining adherents and has led a number of writers to question the more general relationship between medical care and health. Clearly, we can measure the outputs of the medical care system — hospital beds, patients treated, new technology — but how does this relate to health? If health is defined as absence of symptoms of a particular disease, the link is clear. But if a broadened concept of health leads us to reject this pathological definition, the relationship is unclear. The anti-medicine school begins with the failure to establish the link between medical care and health, and suggests that the answer is to move the burden of medical care from the institutionalized health-care system and back to the individual.

One of the most extreme proponents of the antimedicine position is Rick Carlson, who calls for the dissolution of the present medical-care system, demystification of the physician, and a reexamination of the concept of health with emphasis on the ability of individuals to care for themselves. Carlson attacks the professional dominance of medicine, which has served to make patients dependent on a technological, service machine. Illich, chief radical theoretician of the movement, carries the idea a step further, focusing on the iatrogenic effects of the medical-care system. Illich expands the concept of iatrogenesis, which usually refers to medically caused illness such as infections from hospitalization or side effects of clinical intervention, to two broader levels. After arguing that clinical iatrogenesis is becoming the major output of the health system, he considers the impact of overmedicalization on the psychological and cultural environments. The medical-care profession has increasingly seized the role of defining sickness, and has increasingly broadened that to include more and more human activity. The result is that the medical system increasingly dominates all aspects of social life, from family to work and even, at the level of structural iatrogenesis, supplanting religion as a substitute for the humanizing experience of suffering.

Whether the relationship between medical care and health is empty but benign, or iatrogenic, the point remains that the huge investments in medical care have not been demonstrated to produce equal returns in the improvement of health. Two examples may emphasize this point. The Karen Quinlan case is a good example of the tendencies of the present medical system to provide more and more care with less and less results. In addition to the ethical questions about death and dignity the case has raised, perhaps a more relevant problem

---

[a]The so-called "end-of-medicine" or "antimedicine" literature has grown quickly in the last year, and has attracted a lot of attention. The two major contributions are by Illich and Carlson. Ivan Illich, *Medical Nemesis: The Expropriation of Health* (New York: Pantheon Books, 1976); and Rick J. Carlson, *The End of Medicine* (New York: John Wiley & Sons, 1975).

it uncovers is the cost-effectiveness of all such heroic efforts. Would the money and other resources spent there have been better spent, and produced more health, if allocated to providing preventive screening to ghetto infants, or food to the undernourished, or better sanitation facilities to rural communities? Beyond that, who ought to decide what allocation of resources best promotes health?

The second example raising similar questions is in the area of leaping technology, for instance the introduction of computerized axial tomography. This equipment allows more sophisticated diagnosis and observation of body tissue than ever possible. Every hospital and some physicians want one. But its high cost, estimated nationwide at $2.5 billion per year if all demands were filled,[6] raises the real question of whether society can afford such medical technology. Again, the central policy question is one of how to measure and achieve the highest return in health from investment in this technology, and who should decide.

One of the -positive responses by and to the anti-medicine literature has been a revived interest in public or social health. Although in part simply a change in application of the same high technology, as in much of the preventive-health movement, and in multiphasic screening,[7] we are now coming to view disease as a social problem, as a consequence of how people live. Increasing the level of carcinogens in the environment as a by-product of industrialization and urbanization; maldistribution of income; poor dietary habits; indulgence in alcohol, tobacco, and other drugs; and motor vehicles are increasingly the major causes of death and disability.[8] Furthermore, in recent years we have come to think of health as including psychological and interpersonal well-being. This broadening is reflected in recent work toward defining health-status indicators, which have concentrated on the aggregation of individuals' perceptions of their ability to perform normal activities as the basis of the measurements. Health becomes, from this perspective, a social not a scientific problem; a collective, not an individual problem. The point of view of the nineteenth-century father of pathology, Rudolph Virchow, appears more relevant: "Medicine is nothing but a social science. Politics is nothing but medicine on a large scale."[9]

If politics is medicine, medicine is also politics, especially in articulating a concept of health. One important criticism of present government efforts in the health field is that the emphasis in biomedical research has been on the cure of disease, not its prevention. Programs to reduce alcohol consumption, decrease drug use, eliminate or modify cigarette smoking, lower automobile speed limits, and ensure cleaner air might be more effective in reducing health costs than further expenditures on medical care. Leon S. White writes: "We must broaden the search [to improve the public's health] to include studies of the impact of life style on health . . . to ignore [the influence of life style] because it doesn't fit into our current methods and approaches to the analysis of health problems is inexcusable."[10]

The politics of health is especially prone to overstatement of rhetoric, oversimplification of issues and underestimation of costs. The public's lack of sophistication concerning health policy is not surprising given the government's own difficulty in clearly defining its own role and goals in this area. Daniel Moynihan describes the gap between intent and outcome in the area of health policy:

There is in the federal process an illusion of accomplishment. We proposed and passed legislation, signed some bills, set up an agency or two. But one finds afterwards that nothing has actually occurred—something has only been incurred. Years after you thought you had a big program going to solve a particular problem, you discover you have, in fact, nothing.[11]

This scenario of heightened public expectations and limited understanding can lead to rapid public disillusionment and overresponse. The political reality of public budgets and their sensitivity to politics threatens health accomplishments and possibly has begun to seriously erode the public's expectations and the system's own credibility.

The central problem for health policy is that because of the problem of measuring health as opposed to measuring medical services, and because of the vested interest of the medical-care industry in expansion, what passes for health policy appears in reality to be policy designed to deal with the cost, distribution, or access to *sick care,* and these policies really only deal with ways of stimulating and guaranteeing further growth of the medical-care industry without guaranteeing improvements in public health. Regulation of medical care, as practiced today, might have only marginal impact on health, and might as Illich argues lead to a deterioration in the quality of public health.

Clearly, the marginal utility of medical-care expenditures is not infinitely positive. At some point the polity must decide its own limits — but at present, these limits remain undefined and politically, for government and the industry, health remains a growth area.

The Size of the Health-Care Industry

As recently as 1950, total expenditures for health care in the United States amounted to only $12 billion, about $78 per person and 4.6 percent of gross national product.[12] By fiscal 1975, these costs had increased ten-fold to $118.5 billion, representing $550 per person, and a sharply increased 8.3 percent of GNP. If and when some form of national health insurance is enacted, these costs will undoubtedly increase still further and faster.[13]

The sources of increase in health expenditures, and the question of what we are buying, rather than simply the absolute size of the costs, is the major issue of concern. From 1950 to 1975, the increase in health expenditures was $92.7

8

billion. Of this amount, the Social Security Administration reports that $13.9 billion, or 15 percent, is due to increased population, but that $44.9 billion, or 48.4 percent, is due to increases in price, and that the remaining $33.9 billion, or 36.6 percent, is due to increases in utilization and changes in the commodity mix, representing more expensive, if not better, technology. If we further break this 25-year period into a pre- and post-Medicare era, the results are quite startling, as reported in table 1-1. Comparing these two periods, we can see the diminishing impact of population growth on health expenditures, along with the sharply increasing impact of inflation in price increases, and a smaller increase in utilization and technology.

These large increases in health costs are unevenly distributed among the various segments of the health-care industry. Table 1-2 contains aggregate and per-capita expenditures for hospital, physician, and other personal health expenditures for the years 1950, 1965, and 1975. Increasingly, hospital care has absorbed a larger share of personal health-care expenditures, from 35.5 percent in 1950 to 45.2 percent in 1975. Physician costs have declined from 25.5 percent of the total to 21.4 percent, and costs of other services have declined from 38.6 percent to 33.4 percent. This pattern is also evident in the rate of growth in these three categories. Over the 15 years, total personal health-care expenditures grew by 603 percent, but hospital costs increased 892 percent, physician costs 482 percent, and other costs 509 percent. Physicians, often accused of being the central greedy force behind escalating health-care costs, directly account for a small and declining share of those expenditures. Hospitals, on the other hand, account for an increasing share of health expenditures.

Table 1-3 indicates United States health expenditures as a percentage of GNP. Health expenditures as a percentage of GNP increased only 13 percent

Table 1-1

Components of Health-Care Expenditure Change, 1950-75

Source of Increase	1950-75	1950-65	1965-75
	Amount of Increase (in billions)		
Price	44.9	10.2	36.9
Population	13.9	4.9	6.1
Other	33.9	7.9	26.7
Total.	$92.7	$23.0	$69.7
	Percentage Distribution		
Price	48.4	44.3	53.0
Population	15.0	21.5	8.7
Other	36.6	34.2	38.3
Total.	100.0%	100.0%	100.0%

Source: *Social Security Bulletin,* February 1976, p. 13.

Table 1-2
Aggregate and Per-Capita Health Expenditures, by Type

	Aggregate Expenses (in millions)		
	1950	*1965*	*1975*
Hospital	$ 3,698 (35.5%)	$13,152 (39.3%)	$ 46,600 (45.2%)
Physician	2,689 (25.9%)	8,405 (25.1%)	22,100 (21.4%)
Other	4,013 (38.6%)	11,941 (35.6%)	34,500 (33.4%)
Total	10,400 (100.0%)	33,498 (100.0%)	103,200 (100.0%)
	Per Capita		
Hospital	$24.09	$ 66.89	$215.12
Physician	17.52	42.75	102.02
Other	26.14	60.72	159.26
Total	67.75	170.36	476.40
	Percent Change Per Capita		
	50-75	*50-65*	*65-75*
Hospital	892	178	222
Physician	482	144	139
Other	509	132	162
Total	603	151	180

Source: *Social Security Bulletin*, February 1976, p. 12.

between 1950 and 1960, but shot up 38.5 percent between 1960 and 1970, and increased another 15.27 percent to 1975.

Increases in the percentage of GNP devoted to medical care indicate that health expenditures have become relatively more important over time. The Council on Wage and Price Stability reports that health-care costs are rising

Table 1-3
United States Health Expenditures as
Percentage of Gross National Product

Year	Percentage of GNP
1950	4.6
1955	4.6
1960	5.2
1965	5.9
1970	7.2
1975	8.3

Source: *Social Security Bulletin*, February 1976, p. 5.

much more rapidly than the overall rate of inflation, that such expenses are "impacting" the disposable income of every family and that these increasing costs are expected to rise sharply for the foreseeable future.[14] In more concrete terms, the cost of an average stay in the hospital rose from $311 in 1965 to $1,017 in 1975, an increase of 327 percent. Some of the council's other findings are also quite startling:

1. The medical-care services component of the Consumer Price Index rose 10.3 percent in 1975, with hospital service charges rising by 13 percent and physician fees rising by 11.8 percent, compared with 7.7 percent for the CPI's overall service component less medical services.
2. The drugs and prescriptions component of the Consumer Price Index rose 7.4 percent in 1975, a highly unusual rate since in the past these prices have rarely increased more than 1 percent annually.
3. Health expenditures as a percent of our Gross National Product rose to an unprecedented level of 8.3 percent in 1975, up 41 percent from the 5.9 level in 1965.
4. Health-care expenditures have tripled since 1965, up from $39 billion to $119 billion; the 1974 increase of $15 billion was the biggest in our history.[15]

The size of the health-care industry can also be appreciated by examining the number of people employed in that sector, and the value of capital goods invested in health facilities. Since 1950 the number of employees has nearly tripled, from about 1.6 million to over 4.4 million, now representing over 5 percent of the employed population.[16] The United States in 1973 had 7,678 hospitals, with over 1.5 million beds, amounting to 7.4 beds per-thousand population.[17] Nursing homes and related facilities include an additional 28,500 facilities with an additional 1.5 million beds.[18] The total assets of all hospitals in 1973 was almost $50 billion.[19]

The present size and rate of growth of the health industry, when coupled with the cultural impact of health and medical care, define a situation that requires public evaluation of the amount of resources being consumed and the return from those resources. As the portion of total national resources devoted to health climbs toward 10 percent, and as the level of health fails to improve along with it, questions of the optimal allocation of resources arise, and these must be addressed in part by establishing more rational evaluations of costs and benefits, and in part by ensuring that the dollars spent on health are productive.

The Health-Care Market[b]

With the increased scope of federal health-insurance programs, and the

---

[b]This discussion of the health-care market is necessarily brief. See Chapter 6, pp. 107ff, for a more complete discussion.

almost universal coverage of private insurance for the working population, the health-care market has become dominated by a multitude of sellers of services and a few large buyers, a situation economists label *oligopsony*. Health-care expenditures in the United States have increased dramatically both in absolute and relative terms, especially since 1965. Most importantly, with the enactment of Medicare and Medicaid legislation, federal involvement in medical financing has dramatically increased.

Heightened public interest in controlling health-care costs is in part due to the political involvement of government since the Medicare era began in 1965, in contrast to relatively limited governmental costs prior to this legislation. Furthermore, the precedent of government-financed health care for the aged and the poor has led to tremendous interest and discussion of expanding such benefits to additional groups.

Increases in health-care expenditures and especially in the price of health care have been mainly attributed to two major factors, which describe the health-care market:

1. Third party payers who lack incentives to hold down costs, which are in turn passed on through increased premiums to consumers
2. Non-competitive nature of the market, and the inelasticity of supply

These have, in effect, changed the nature of the health-care market, and shaped the problems of regulation and cost control we now face.

Third-Party Payers

Traditional market theory holds that the price of a commodity acts as a control on the amount demanded. As price rises, consumers will purchase less; as it falls, they will purchase more. Increasingly in the health field, the availability of health insurance, which usually amounts to prepayment of health costs,[20] has lowered the direct cost to the consumer at the point of delivery, removed the price constraint, and resulted in increased consumption of health resources.

Table 1-4 presents the sources of personal health expenditures at point of service for three years: 1950, 1965, and 1975. Especially for hospital care, direct payment by patients has decreased significantly over this quarter-century. For hospitals, the direct share has declined from 34.2 percent in 1950 to 8 percent in 1975, while the portion of the hospital bill paid by private insurance has increased from 16.5 percent to 35.8 percent, and the public share has increased from 16.5 percent to 35.8 percent. For physician care, direct costs have dropped dramatically from 84.8 percent to 34.5 percent, while both private insurance and public funding have increased. The consumer still pays a large share of other costs (primarily dentist, eyeglasses, and drugs) directly, but insurance and public monies now cover an increasing share of those as well. By 1975 total direct payments for all personal health-care services amounted

Table 1–4
Percentage Distribution of Personal Health-Care Expenditures by Source of Payment

	1950	1965	1975
Hospital			
Direct	34.2%	18.5%	8.0%
Insurance	16.5	41.7	35.8
Public	45.7	37.5	55.0
Physician			
Direct	84.8	63.2	34.5
Insurance	10.0	30.4	39.0
Public	4.9	6.3	26.5
Other			
Direct	88.8	82.3	64.5
Insurance	–	2.0	5.9
Public	7.0	12.6	27.3

Source: *Social Security Bulletin*, February 1976, p. 18.

to $33.6 billion, only 32.5 percent of total personal health costs as opposed to 68.3 percent in 1950.

As the percentage of expenses paid by consumers directly has dropped, the portion of the population covered by health insurance has increased. The Social Security Administration estimates that by December 31, 1974, 79.9 percent of the under-65 population had private insurance for hospital care, 78.3 percent for surgical care, 77.5 percent for in-hospital physician care, 77.5 percent for x-ray and lab exams, 62.3 percent for office visits, and 73.2 percent for drugs. Only 17.4 percent had dental coverage, although coverage for these services was growing rapidly. Most over-65 persons are covered by Medicare, and an additional 5 to 10 percent are covered by state Medicaid programs.[21] Estimates by the Health Insurance Association of America, a private group, are even higher.[22]

There is an unmistakable correlation between the growth of health-insurance coverage and the rise in health costs. As the share of hospital costs paid out-of-pocket has declined from 34.0 percent to 8.0 percent from 1950 to 1975, the total hospital bill has increased from $3.7 billion to $46.6 billion, and has increased its share of total health expenditures from 35.5 percent to 45.2 percent. By removing the price constraint on the use of health resources, the third-party effect has changed the behavior of patients and resulted in a basic change in the health-care market. This change is magnified by the fact that the major third-party payers are able to pass price and cost increases along to the consumer in the form of higher premiums, and hence have only minimal incentives to control costs and utilization. This is especially true because the return on invested premiums is a major source of the net income of private insurers, and higher income here becomes a goal regardless of eventual claim costs. The clientele of the health-insurance industry tends to be providers, who want more dollars, rather than the consumers, who ultimately pay the bill. To the extent that health financing bureaucracies, both public and private, are captured by the sellers, the problem of control of the system becomes unsolvable.

Supply of Health Care

On the other side of the equation, the providers of health care comprise what is often referred to as a nonsystem.[c] Thousands of independent providers supply uncoordinated, maldistributed, and inefficient services. Physician location, distribution of specialists, and the number of hospital beds defy rational planning. Professionalism is used as a means of controlling access to the market, and to prevent or delay innovations in organization, such as physician assistants or health-maintenance organizations, which would provide potential savings in costs and improvements in health care.

Victor Fuchs has called attention to the particular structure of the medical-care industry, which contrasts with the model of actively competing, profit-seeking firms. The normal rationale that the desire for profits (and fear of loss) will best guarantee efficiency, appropriate price and rate of output, and fair returns does not hold in this situation.

Nonprofit operations are the rule in the hospital field; there are severe restrictions on entry and competition in medical practice; and advertising and patent control dominate the market for drugs.[23]

Although doctors have often invoked the cliches of free enterprise to justify laissez-faire and the status quo, the nonmarket nature of much activity in this field is apparent and appears to justify (even for many economists) governmental intervention. In fact, government efforts to increase competition, for example, through changes in licensure and in the generic labeling of drugs, have been fiercely resisted in the name of the quality of care and the doctor-patient relationship. Governmental intervention through licensure has been long accepted but the precedent and its implications have been resisted. As H.E. Frech III recently noted, health care "has been heavily regulated for many years and may be the most regulated sector of the economy."[24]

Frech suggests two explanatory hypotheses for the politics of regulation:

1. *Consumer protection hypothesis:* regulation benefits the consumer by reducing monopolistic exploitation, compensating for market imperfection.

---

[c]See Chapters 5 and 6 for more discussion of these issues.

2. *Producer-protection hypotheses:* governmental regulation serves producer interests, largely by reducing competition.

In accepting the latter hypothesis Frech concludes "the evidence seems quite strong that medical care regulation can be characterized in this way, and that it has often aided providers, either by directly reducing competition or by aiding private activities of producers that have anti-competitive effects."[25]

Increasing medical manpower by increasing the number of medical students or increased training and use of physician extenders or paraprofessionals have been proposed, but the proposals fail to deal with concomitant problems of continuing medical specialization (i.e., the shortage of primary care physicians) and maldistribution.[26] Policies that deal with the former, but the latter, problems are doomed to failure. In criticizing these policy proposals, which he characterized as "market reforms," Robert Alford suggests that these reforms do not seriously damage any present medical interests.[27] He continues: "This pluralistic balancing of costs and benefits successfully defends the funding, powers, and resources of the producing institutions against any basic structural change."[28] Alford suggests that corporate rationalizers including hospital administrators, medical schools, government health planners, public health agencies, and researchers are interested in breaking down the professional monopoly of physicians over the production and distribution of health care.[29]

Alford also suggests a second reformist thrust that might help control health-care costs. Bureaucratic reformers blame market competition for the defects of the system and call for increased administrative regulation and government financing and control of health care. They are concerned with changing the health-care delivery system by coordinating fragmented services, instituting planning, and extending public funding. Although in the long run such changes may help control health-care costs, new mechanisms and methods of health-care delivery are long-term approaches, which in turn may be more easily spurred by cost-containment efforts rather than the reverse.[30]

Federal government efforts to control health-care costs are of relatively recent vintage, stemming mostly from open-ended costs in the Medicare program. Earlier exhortations and controls in the search for a wage-price policy that would reconcile full employment, reasonable price stability, and free economic institutions, have included monetary fiscal policies, guideposts, moral suasion, a productivity principle, threats of *ad hoc* government pressure, 'ground rules', inflation alerts, 'New Economic Policy', and finally President Nixon's wage-price controls. Only the latter seem to have had a clear impact since World War II. Federal "price fighters" have only recently begun to use and to explore the possible leverage of the enormous federal health budget expenditures to try to effectuate a degree of relative price stability. In general, wage-price policies since Truman have been encouraged by a number of factors, including the goal of full employment, wars (which have generated wide oscillations in economic performance), and elections. The assumption is that many labor and product markets are characterized by non-competitive conditions and that such monopoly power must be countervailed to prevent inflation and the resulting economic and social instability.

Unfortunately, past efforts have been flawed by several problems that also complicate and frustrate efforts to control health-care costs:

1. A consistent failure of and rules governing wage-price policy
2. An inability to achieve an even-handed treatment of wages and prices
3. The failure to develop standards that are comprehensive, equitable and succinctly precise[31]

Wages and prices in the health field are dealt with as in other sectors of the economy, but, with an important exception. With professional monopolists dominating the system they have captured a preponderance of the pecuniary rewards. On the other hand, less-skilled employees have only recently begun to organize collectively to obtain a fairer return for their labors. The inequalities and glaring differences in the wages of doctors, nurses, and other health personnel is mirrored in concomitant societal and personal differences in status, which have frustrated many health professionals, including nurses and pharmacists.

Finally, there are no clear standards or measures of outputs or performance that are comprehensive, equitable, and succinctly precise. Policy, where it does exist (e.g., efforts to control drug costs as discussed by Fulda),[32] is discrete, disjointed (in its inapplication to all of society), and of questionable equity, with no clear-cut conception of the public good or public interest beyond vague legislative rhetoric.[33] Standards are only iterated on the basis of political pressure—public and interest-group outcries and the political sensitivities and public-interest perceptions of elected officials.

Thus, rather than facing a pure market situation in dealing with health care, we instead face a market with these characteristics:

1. The supply of health care is constrained by artificial restrictions on entry and other devices.
2. The consumers of health care increasingly lack control, through price, over supply.
3. Bureaucratization of the payment and hospital segments of the industry and disorganization of physician supply make the regulatory problem increasingly complex.
4. Increased government, especially federal government, involvement in the health-care market

These factors shape a situation, described and analyzed in the following chapters, perhaps unique in the American economy, and perhaps not amenable to present regulation and control approaches.

Conclusion

Fuchs suggests that "because payment for medical care is increasingly regarded as a collective responsibility, it is natural and appropriate that there should be collective expressions of concern."[34] The cliche "he that pays the piper calls the tune" has increasingly become the reality in the health-care field. Government effort to increase the marginal returns on health-care expenditures has resulted in more and more specifications on how funds can be used and what results are expected. Efforts that return easily measurable benefits are easier to rationalize with elected officials and with the public, who ultimately pay the bill.

In emphasizing the necessity for choice Fuchs concludes that "we cannot have all the health or all the medical care that we would like to have."[35] His caveats are a useful preface to these chapters, which attempt to break new ground. "Some health care problems defy 'solution.' At most one can hope for understanding, adjustment, amelioration."[36]

There is probably no need to reiterate the difficulty of resolving the problems dealt with in this book or the controversial nature of the subject. Almost every contributor will reiterate it in her or his chapter. Although some health-care problems do, as Fuchs noted, defy "solution," and we clearly cannot have all the health or all the medical care that we would like to have, it appears that adjustment and amelioration of our present situation must come (and has in the health policy area come) through the political process. It is clear, as Walter McClure later suggests, that "the structure and incentives producing the problems in our present medical care system are very strong and deep-rooted."[37] Our modest efforts in this volume seek to help build understanding by considering the implementation of present policy, efforts to control health-care costs, and the politics and future of health-care policy. Hopefully, we can contribute to the development of a national health policy in America that will further a better and healthier society.

Part II

Federal Health-Control Policy: Three Cases

2

The Social Security Administration and Medicare: A Strategy of Implementation

Judith M. Feder

Before July 1965, the Social Security Administration (SSA) was an independent, relatively noncontroversial agency responsible for pension and disability payments to eligible individuals. Since that date, SSA has become a powerful participant in the health-care system, and the focus of political pressure from inside the executive branch, organized interest groups, and Congress. This change is largely the result of SSA's responsibility for Medicare implementation. In coping with it, SSA has demonstrated three characteristics: (1) a commitment to remaining primarily a distributor of welfare benefits, (2) a desire to avoid controversy and have operations run smoothly, and (3) an effort to secure autonomous control over its program and survival as an independent agency.

Theoretically, SSA could have acted very differently in administering Medicare. As the largest third-party payer in the health-care field, SSA could have emphasized its health responsibility more than its benefit task. Officials might then have taken a very active and aggressive attitude toward the health industry, defining health goals and requiring compliance. But none of these descriptions apply. The history of SSA's administration of hospital insurance illustrates instead how the opposite characteristics have intertwined to shape Medicare policy.

That SSA approached Medicare implementation this way rather than any other is not because officials did not know or care about the impact of their policies on the medical-care system. On the contrary, they believed that the power of the medical-care establishment in the American political system would have doomed any other approach to failure and federal health insurance to extinction. This chapter cannot test that judgment, which may well have been correct. But the fact that bureaucracies make such judgments and the costs they entail have significant implications for Medicare and further federal health-insurance programs.

An earlier version of this chapter was published by Spectrum Research, Inc., as the final chapter of *The Character and Implications of SSA's Administration of Medicare.* Research and preparation of that monograph were supported by Grant No. 10-P-57693/8-01 from the Social Security Administration to the Policy Center, Inc. Patrick O'Donoghue, M.D., president of the Policy Center, Inc., and co-director of this project, was largely responsible for developing the analytical framework based on the research findings, and for elaborating several of the policy implications. Under his leadership, valuable contributions were also made by participants in the project's second ad hoc advisory group meeting: Rick Carlson, Clark Havighurst, Ted Marmor, and Roger Noll.

SSA's Administration of Medicare

Primacy of Benefit Task

Perhaps the clearest evidence of SSA's decision to remain a benefit payer has been the agency's subordination of quality enforcement to its benefit-payment task. SSA's responsibility for hospital quality derived from two requirements in the Medicare law: first, that hospitals meet certain quality criteria to be eligible for Medicare funds; and second, the specific requirement that hospitals have a committee to review and evaluate their delivery of services, that is, a hospital utilization review committee.[1] Implementing these requirements presented SSA with a choice. Because the law deemed all hospitals accredited by the industry's Joint Commission on Accreditation of Hospitals (JCAH) eligible for Medicare participation, the agency's quality criteria would apply only to unaccredited hospitals.[2] These were primarily small, rural hospitals, many of which health professionals considered inadequately staffed, poorly equipped, and fundamentally unsafe. Requiring professionally acceptable quality of Medicare hospitals meant denying these hospitals certification, putting many of them out of business. Allowing these hospitals to participate, on the other hand, meant perpetuating inadequate hospitals with Medicare funds.

Facing this choice, SSA saw its major responsibility as "paying for care where people get care," that is, simply paying benefits; and they attempted to develop regulations accordingly. But they were pushed toward quality oversight by the Public Health Service (PHS) and some professional representatives on the Health Insurance Benefits Advisory Council (HIBAC), with whom the law required they consult. PHS and their supporters on the council saw in Medicare an opportunity to improve the quality of hospital care.[a]

SSA did not accept this objective. "PHS wanted the millenium," recalled a senior Medicare official. "We were concerned with having a program on July 1, 1966." With that concern in mind, SSA officials were willing to compromise with quality advocates. They promulgated relatively high standards, which everyone felt many hospitals would be unable to meet, but allowed considerable leeway in determining compliance—a requirement of full compliance with quality standards.[3] In other words, hospitals falling short of the standards could receive Medicare funds. With this approach SSA could certify most hospitals

---

[a]This issue is discussed in detail in *The Character and Implications of SSA's Administration of Medicare,* Denver: Spectrum Research, Inc., 1975, Chapter II. It is based primarily on minutes of the Health Insurance Benefits Advisory Council (HIBAC), Meeting 1: Session 2, November 13, 1965, pp. 14–16; John W. Cashman, M.D., and Beverlee A. Myers, M.P.H., F.A.P.H.A., "Medicare Standards of Services in a New Program—Licensure, Certification, Accreditation," *American Journal of Public Health,* 57 (July 1967) especially p. 1113; and personal interviews with PHS and SSA officials.

pay benefits, and avoid both aggressive quality enforcement and overt support of substandard hospital care.

Implementation of the law's specific requirement for utilization review followed a similar course. Although members of the medical profession advocated utilization review as a means of quality and cost control, this was a new concept in 1965 and few committees actually existed. Including it in the law as a requirement for hospital participation made SSA responsible for establishing a new professional practice, a task the agency was loath to undertake. Accordingly, they left the hospitals to determine their own approaches to review; did not establish the time criteria for review that the law intended; delegated primary oversight authority to fiscal intermediaries rather than to the agencies responsible for determining hospital compliance with the law, the state health departments; and undertook only minimal supervision of both. Reliance on intermediaries rather than state agencies essentially removed utilization review from the certification arena and substituted encouragement and persuasion for quality regulation.[b] The implications of this approach and the strength of SSA's bias became apparent when the agency first became concerned about program costs. Rather than enforce utilization review to ensure provision of and payment for services consistent with the law, the agency chose to ignore it. Instead they authorized their fiscal agents, the intermediaries, simply to deny payment for inappropriate claims.[4] This policy created a potential problem for beneficiaries, for claim denial applies retroactively and therefore lacks the advance notice and due process that utilization review required.[5] It was, however, consistent with SSA's preference for determining the validity of claims for benefits rather than reviewing medical practice.

Avoidance of Controversy

SSA's resistance to becoming an enforcer of quality also reflects the second of the agency's fundamental characteristics — its avoidance of controversy and desire for smooth operations. Reinforcing its predilection to act as it had always acted was SSA's continual effort to compromise competing political interests and pressures. Having demonstrated their agility in this game in the

---

[b]These decisions are described in *Character and Implications,* Chapter V. It is based primarily on interviews with SSA officials; HIBAC minutes, memoranda, and consultant work-group meetings, November and December 1965; "Responsibilities of Intermediaries and State Agencies in the Area of Provider Utilization Practices," staff memorandum for HIBAC, HIBAC Agenda Book, April 30–May 1, 1966; "Medicare and Medicaid; Problems, Issues and Alternatives," Report of the staff to the Finance Committee, U.S. Senate, Committee Print, 91st Cong., 1st session, February 9, 1970, p. 106 ff.

legislative bargaining that led to the law's enactment,[c] Medicare's architects, most of whom came from SSA, approached implementation from the same perspective. They believed the cooperation of the health-care industry was essential to the successful start and continuing existence of their program and made its achievement a primary goal in 1965. The same strategy of consensus and compromise, rather than conflict, characterized SSA's approach to certification, reimbursement, and innovation throughout their administration of Medicare.

With respect to hospital certification and utilization review, officials had no doubt that they had more to lose than to gain from a policy of active quality enforcement.[d] To fulfill Medicare's promise, they considered it essential that enough hospitals be certified to guarantee that all the elderly had access to care. No one knew for certain how many people would seek care – and how many beds would be necessary – on Medicare's first day. President Lyndon Johnson, who had identified himself with the Medicare program, made it top priority that anyone seeking a Medicare-financed bed in July 1966 be able to find one. As one official recalled, there was great concern that too literal an application of quality standards would mean too few beds. Even where this was not the case, officials believed that the elderly and the nation expected Medicare to pay for care where the elderly generally received it. Stringent requirements for hospital participation would disrupt patterns of hospital use, leaving the elderly disappointed and the nation unimpressed. Furthermore, Medicare officials felt that unless the people and institutions that had to deliver care cooperated with government administrators, getting care to the people and ensuring the program's survival would be fraught with difficulty. Achieving that cooperation meant avoiding the threat to professional autonomy and, in many cases, to institutions' financial viability that denial of certification would pose.

In view of the overall configuration of political interests, SSA decided to avoid policies that would close hospitals. This perspective shaped SSA's enforcement as well as its promulgation of standards over the years. Officials explicitly defined their role as an educational rather than a policing responsibility and regarded termination for noncompliance as a weapon too powerful to use very often. Pushed by quality-conscious PHS officials, SSA did in fact terminate some hospitals. Ever cautious, SSA kept tight central control over

---

[c]For Medicare's legislative history, see Peter A. Corning, *The Evolution of Medicare . . . From Idea to Law,* HEW, SSA, ORS, Research Report Number 29, Washington, U.S., Government Printing Office, 1969; Richard Harris, *A Sacred Trust,* Baltimore: Penguin Books, Inc., 1969 (first published in 1966); Theodore R. Marmor with the assistance of Jan S. Marmor, *The Politics of Medicare,* Chicago: Aldine Publishing Company, 1970.

[d]This account is developed in chapters II and V of *Character and Implications.* It is based primarily on personal interviews with HEW, SSA, and PHS officials and sources in footnote a, and reference note 3, page 233.

termination actions, sought approval from Congressional delegations, and never acted against a hospital unless they were sure they could win. The result was to terminate far fewer hospitals than an assessment of actual compliance with the law would require.[6]

SSA further revealed its concern with smooth operations in this area by accepting the existing political configuration and by resisting consumer advocates' attempts to alter it. In the view of SSA officials, the "educational" approach to quality has been effective and valuable; they believe they press hospitals as far as politically possible and cite congressional support of providers as indicative of political constraints.[e] Although there is validity to this point of view, SSA's interest in maintaining a low profile on quality enforcement has caused the agency to resist the takeover of full-quality responsibility from the JCAH and to oppose consumer involvement in the certification process.

In 1969 HIBAC sharply criticized Medicare's reliance on JCAH accreditation to ensure quality care and advocated appropriate changes in the Medicare law.

Initially, Medicare's reliance on JCAH accreditation standards and certification procedures helped the new Federal program win the acceptance and support of the health professions and was beneficial to both the government and the health professions. The Council believes, however, that it is inappropriate to continue statutory delegation to a private agency of all the Government's authority to safeguard quality of care paid for by a government program. The authority to establish policy on minimum quality should be retained by the Government. Quality standards under Medicare should not be controlled by a private agency's standards. Furthermore, the power of oversight and assurance that standards are applied adequately in individual situations should and must remain within both the responsibility and authority of the Government.[7]

Although Medicare officials worked with JCAH to upgrade its standards, HEW never initiated legislation to expand its authority over hospital quality.[8] A consumer law suit, however, led Congress to enact amendments in 1972 that authorized HEW surveys of accredited hospitals in response to complaints and on a sample basis and removed the JCAH ceiling on Medicare standards.[f] SSA has undertaken the required surveys, but, as always, fear of political repercussions has made the agency move slowly and cautiously.

SSA took a similar position on public disclosure of hospital surveys for certification. Over the agency's objections, in 1972 Congress required SSA to

---

[e]Interviews with SSA officials. Congressional passage of the Burleson Amendment of 1970, which waived 24-hour nursing requirements for small, rural hospitals, was particularly important in restraining terminations. See *Character and Implications,* Chapter II.

[f]For a discussion of the law suit, see "Suit Challenges Delegation of Medicare's Standards to JCAH," *Hospital Practice* (February 1972), p. 186 ff. Amendments were in P.L. 92-603, Sec. 244, enacted October 30, 1972.

make these surveys public.[g] Although SSA has complied with the law, some officials report inadequate publicity of the disclosure provisions. Another program official denied this charge, pointing to the agency's effort to inform district offices and contractors of the new requirement. But asked whether SSA had also informed beneficiaries of the available information, this official said they had not; perhaps, she said, a "flaw" in their efforts.[9]

SSA's reactions to the 1972 changes in certification reveal its reluctance to attract increased public attention and political pressure. To SSA, new responsibilities and expanded consumer participation mean disruption of the procedures and relationships to which the agency has become accustomed; in sum, unwelcome change.

SSA's desire to avoid controversy by obtaining and maintaining hospital cooperation is equally apparent with respect to payment policy. At the start of Medicare, no issue received greater attention that the development of principles for provider reimbursement.[h] Over the years of legislative consideration, government officials believed that a consensus had been reached on payment procedures, and they had promised to follow established industry practices. But after enactment, the consensus disappeared as hospitals sought to acquire the most favorable payment arrangements they could. To the extent that these arrangements would have exceeded estimates on which Medicare financing was based, agreeing to them would force the agency to seek a tax increase from Congress. SSA thus faced opposing pressures, from providers on the one hand, and Congress, in particular the Senate Finance Committee, on the other.[10]

SSA's response was to try to compromise these competing interests, making enough concessions to satisfy the hospitals without necessitating a tax increase. The difference between this negotiated arrangement and one based on SSA bureaucratic definition of the role Medicare *ought* to play in hospital financing is apparent in comparing the final regulations on reimbursement with the initial proposals of SSA staff. Based on their conception of the public interest and a desire to avoid costs in excess of estimates, officials in SSA's Bureau of Health Insurance (BHI) developed policy recommendations closely restricting hospital reimbursement to patient-care costs, and requiring a technically sophisticated method of calculation intended to ensure accuracy (RCCAC). Their intent was to ensure that the program paid only its appropriate share of a hospital's total costs and to avoid the potential for health-cost inflation and diminished community control over hospitals that reimbursement in excess of costs could produce.[11] Clearly aware of this possibility, BHI officials sought reimbursement procedures that would avoid its realization.

---

[g]P.L. 92-603, Sec. 249C. SSA position discussed in "Top Secret" at SSA, Why?" *Hospital Practice* (February 1972), pp. 195–196. Supported by personal interviews with SSA officials.

[h]Elaborated in *Character and Implications,* Chapter III.

Although it is questionable whether any payment system based on costs can avoid inflationary consequences, there is no question that the reimbursement principles first developed by BHI meant smaller increases in hospital cash flow than did the principles finally adopted. The agency moved from its initial recommendations in an effort to assuage hospital discontent and, in so doing, contributed to the outcome they had hoped to avoid.[i] Holding on to much of their payment formula in spite of hospital opposition, officials made concessions on allocation and depreciation and awarded a 2 percent plus factor, all of which contributed significantly to hospital net income. The reason for these concessions was the belief, even on the part of officials who had developed the earlier proposals, that without hospital cooperation, smooth implementation of the entire Medicare program would be jeopardized, to the detriment of the agency and its beneficiaries. Officials believed the hospitals would go along with whatever rules the agency promulgated. "But there's a real difference," said a senior official, "in launching a program with the help of the hospitals as opposed to against them." Accordingly, SSA struck a bargain with the hospitals and gained cooperation.[12]

Maintaining that bargain, without increasing or decreasing concessions, became SSA's political objective on reimbursement. Again officials believed there was more to lose than to gain from reopening controversial questions; 7,000 hospitals could make considerable political uproar. One program official stated the Commissioner's guiding principle: "The hospitals can ask for more; but the government cannot offer less."[13] At an operating level, this strategy was supported by bureaucratic conservatism, a desire to stick to procedures already established. Evidence of these concerns comes both from what SSA did and did not do after negotiating reimbursement with the hospitals in 1965-66.

Through the end of the Johnson administration, there was very little reconsideration of reimbursement policy. Indicative of the agency's primary concern with administrative smoothness was their initiation of a streamlined, regularized system of payment (PIP); at the same time they ignored comments from the field and their general counsel on excessive reimbursement.[j] As awareness of rising costs called public attention to their payment system, SSA responded by proposing that Congress authorize them to experiment with incentives for efficiency in reimbursement and to tie depreciation to evaluations

---

[i]For increases in hospital cash flow, see Karen Davis, "Hospital Costs and the Medicare Program," *Social Security Bulletin* (August 1973), especially pp. 20-21.

[j]Discussed in *Character and Implications,* Chapter IV. In particular, see discussion of problems in 1967-68 in "Lengthy Delays in Settling the Costs of Health Services Furnished Under Medicare," SSA, DHEW Report to the Congress by the Comptroller General January 23, 1971, pp. 23-29; and "Administration of Federal Health Programs," Hearings before the Subcommittee of the Committee on Government Operations, House of Representatives, 91/1, Part 1, pp. 79-80. Supported by personal interviews with SSA officials.

of hospital capital expenditures by local planning agencies.[14] SSA officials had little confidence in these proposals[k] but were anxious to appear responsive. Congress reinforced SSA's existing reimbursement policy by rejecting the planning amendment, and, although they authorized reimbursement experimentation, neither Congress nor SSA perceived it as an instrument of comprehensive policy review.

Officials responsible for experimentation were highly sceptical that payment changes would increase hospital efficiency and lower program costs. In 1967 the official who was placed in charge of the experiments, Irwin Wolkstein, made these comments on the subject:

It should be understood that the potential for economy through financial rewards and deterrents is limited. There are many motivations and factors in a complex hospital other than maximizing net operating income from third parties. For one thing, contributions from the community at large, as from specific donors, may sometimes be induced by almost the opposite of economy of operation. The success of a hospital in its administration may be measured not merely by hospital efficiency but also by the completeness of hospital facilities, the fame of its staff, and the wealth of its patients. None of these is necessarily highly correlated with efficiency. . . .[15]

Along with their general questions about incentives and efficiency, officials were extremely doubtful about hospitals' willingness to experiment. The amendment did not require hospital participation in experiments; it simply allowed it. What hospital, officials asked, would choose a reimbursement scheme in which it might lose money? Although Medicare officials raised this question in later years, Congress failed to address it. The result, BHI officials believe, was to render experimentation meaningless.[16]

As a result, the experimental program was a low priority in SSA. Rather than develop formal and specific requests for proposals, through which government usually solicits private research, SSA published general guidelines for experiments and awaited ideas from the private sector. SSA described its "strategy" as

designed to tap the best reservoir of ideas for reimbursement incentives believed to have been already developed by the health services industry and ready for implementation with little or no additional attention.[17]

Speaking less diplomatically, one might say SSA simply issued a challenge to its critics: "If you've got such good ideas, where are they?"

Five years after Congress authorized experiments, SSA had implemented only five proposals. SSA attributed these admittedly meager results to the

---

[k]Officials' doubts about the planning process are described in detail in *Character and Implications,* Chapter IV. The experimental provision became Section 402, HR 12080, Social Security Amendments of 1967.

failure of the private sector to produce the expected projects, the unwillingness of hospitals to risk losing money, and hospitals' "misunderstanding" of the experimental program. Hospitals, officials said, saw experiments as a way "to achieve changes in Medicare reimbursement that would improve the financial position of hospitals, i.e., changes that would tend to increase costs rather than contain or reduce them."[1]

Having struck a bargain on reimbursement in 1965-66, Medicare officials had no intention of allowing hospitals to use experiments to attain financial advantages the agency had already turned down. Hence SSA insisted that experiments identify, measure, and evaluate contributions to efficiency, and rejected any proposal that would cost, after a brief period, more than the ongoing reimbursement approach. With no initiatives on SSA's part, a cautious response to proposals of others, and congressional unwillingness to require hospital participation, this experimentation produced little information of use to policy making. It succeeded, however, in deferring any serious reconsideration of Medicare's reimbursement formula.

Additional evidence of SSA's commitment to that formula and attentiveness to political pressure has been SSA's policy toward group-practice prepayment plans (GPPPs). Encouragement of this innovation in medical organization, characterized by capitation rather than fee-for-service payment, was prominent in public discussion of increased efficiency in Medicare reimbursement. But SSA made few adjustments of its payment principles, devised for the fee-for-service system, to accommodate GPPPs. In spite of GPPP protestations and claims of sympathy by SSA officials, SSA refused to allow advance capitation, and instead required retroactive cost calculations by prepayment plans. In 1966 SSA was preoccupied with arrangements for the majority of medical-care providers and unwilling to disrupt them for unconventional approaches to medical organization with weak political backing.[m] HEW officials who later sought to use SSA's experimentation authority to encourage development of GPPPs, by then called

---

[1]"Status of Program Experimentation in the Bureau of Health Insurance," Staff Memorandum for HIBAC, November 28, 1972, pp. 6-7; Officials' attitudes are discussed in detail in *Character and Implications,* Chapter IV, and are based largely on personal interviews.

[m]GPPP-SSA conflicts are explored in detail in *Character and Implications,* Chapter IV. It is based on interviews with interest groups and SSA officials; HIBAC minutes, VIII, April 30-May 1, 1966; XIV, January 7-8, 1967; "Tying Health Insurance Beneficiaries to Group Practice Prepayment Plans," October 1965, discussed in "Experimentation for Prepaying Organizations to Provide Medical Services—Section 402 of the Social Security Act Amendments of 1967," memo from Office of the General Counsel to Mr. Irwin Wolkstein, Division of Policy and Standards, BHI, May 28, 1971, p. 2; Appendix B in "Status of Program Experimentation," Staff Memorandum for HIBAC, November 28, 1972; Howard West, "Group Practice Prepayment Plans in the Medicare Program," *American Journal of Public Health* 59:4 (April 1969), pp. 624-629; H.F. Newman, "The Impact of Medicare on GPPPs," *American Journal of Public Health* 59:4 (April 1969), pp. 629-634; H.F. Newman, "Medicare and the Comprehensive Health Cooperative of Puget Sound," *Bulletin of the New York Academy of Medicine,* 44 (November 1968), pp. 1321-1323; and R.J. Erikson, "The Impact of Medicare on a Group Practice Prepayment Plan," *Bulletin of the New York Academy of Medicine,* 44 (November 1969), pp. 1312-1320.

Health Maintenance Organizations (HMOs), found SSA's attitude "the biggest sticking point. Their concern is that if you open up the trust fund for incentive reimbursement, particularly to develop HMO's, you're opening it up for a real raid."[18]

Faced with the attempts by a new, and Republican, administration to review and alter policy in 1969, SSA continued to protect its agreement with the hospitals from disruption. Notable examples are its objection to HEW's elimination of the 2 percent-plus, its replacement of the 2 percent factor with the 8-½ percent nursing differential; its reluctance to eliminate allocations options; and its opposition to the withdrawal of current financing and to development of preadmission utilization review.[n] Although positions on these issues were also a product of SSA's assertion of autonomy, they reflected the agency's consistent rule of thumb: where industry discontent would cost more politically than would be gained from reducing program expenditures, stick with the deal you have.

Autonomy and Survival

SSA's approach to policy making did not mean the absence of concern with rising hospital costs. Rather, it defined the limits within which SSA undertook cost-control action. Although some officials within SSA had been concerned from Medicare's beginning about the cost implications of reimbursement concessions, these implications became an agency problem only when increases aroused political discussion and posed a threat to SSA control over Medicare and possible future national health-insurance plans. This occurred in the early Nixon years, with attention in the Administration and Congress to the "health-care crisis" and proposals for national health insurance. Also, during these years, the Senate Finance Committee publicly criticized Medicare's administration as largely responsible for skyrocketing program costs.[19] As costs and program growth have stimulated these and other challenges to SSA's performance, the agency has demonstrated its third outstanding characteristic — an effort to secure its autonomy and survival.

On the cost issue, officials at the top of the Medicare hierarchy have been primarily concerned with warding off attacks on their performance. Accordingly they proposed to solve cost problems by shifting to prospective reimbursement, an approach for which there was widespread support in principle and little agreement in practice.[20] At lower levels in the hierarchy, within BHI, officials had a different perspective. They felt program costs escaping their grasp and saw support in the political environment for doing something about it. Although

---

[n]Personal interviews with officials in HEW, SSA, OMB. Developed in detail in *Character and Implications*, Chapters VI and VII.

these officials believed the only way to restrain hospital expenditures was to reduce reimbursement's unlimited cash flow to individual hospitals,[21] their acceptance of the agency's political strategy severely constrained their policy options. Although they occasionally proposed highly restrictive measures in staff memoranda to HIBAC,[22] they did not seriously pursue them.[23] Instead they attempted to control program costs by eliminating blatant abuse of reimbursement provisions, closing obvious and costly loopholes, and preventing further "rip-offs."

The clearest example of the first cost-control strategy was SSA's response in 1969 to hospitals' manipulation of reimbursement provisions for accelerated depreciation. These provisions made it possible, for example, to boost hospital asset value through resale, causing Medicare to pay depreciation again and again at increasing rates. With the support of the General Accounting Office, the Senate Finance Committee, and the House Ways and Means Committee, BHI altered its regulations and reduced these abuses.° Both BHI's definition of the problem and satisfaction with its resolution reflect officials' compromise between concern with provider cooperation and the achievement of cost control. Handling abuses of accelerated depreciation entailed no reconsideration of the appropriateness of reimbursement for depreciation and capital in general, an area in which SSA had made concessions to hospital demands in 1966. In fact, the changes reinforced the legitimacy of depreciation payments used for capital purposes by distinguishing these from the abuse being eliminated. Second, BHI officials prided themselves on having been able to accomplish a change with relatively little political uproar. They perceived the measure as an unequivocal success.[24]

Another area where SSA made a change in reimbursement was in eliminating the options for calculating the portion of hospital expenditures allocated to Medicare beneficiaries. Options were included in the initial reimbursement formula as a concession to hospital claims that the BHI-advocated method, generally regarded as the most accurate, was more sophisticated than they could implement. The opportunity that this presented for hospitals to select the method of calculation that brought them the greatest revenue was recognized but ignored in Medicare's early years.[25] In spite of awareness, and some concern, that hospitals were taking advantage of this opportunity, SSA was reluctant to

---

°Discussed in detail in *Character and Implications,* Chapter VI. It is based on interviews with SSA officials; "Medicare and Medicaid; Problems, Issues, and Alternatives," Report of the staff to the Finance Committee, U.S. Senate, Committee Print, 91st Cong., 1st session, February 9, 1970; HIBAC minutes, XXX, January 10, 1970. "Social Security Amendments of 1970," Report of the Committee on Ways and Means on HR 17550 (91-1096), May 14, 1970, pp. 64–65; "Payments to Hospitals and Extended Care Facilities for Depreciation Expense Under the Medicare Program," B-142983, SSA, DHEW, Report to the Committee on Finance, U.S. Senate, by the Comptroller General of the United States, August 1970.

deny it to them, particularly after HEW removed the 2 percent-plus factor in 1969.[26] Again through the combined effort of BHI staff and the Senate Finance Committee, the options were finally removed in 1971.[27] The greater difficulty of this change as compared with that on accelerated depreciation further reflects SSA's avoidance of controversy.

SSA's simultaneous concern with avoiding controversy and controlling runaway program costs had two further implications: first, SSA enthusiasm for cost-control action outside the Medicare framework for which they would not have to take the political heat; and, second, within the Medicare framework, a preference for restriction over innovation. BHI responded to the introduction of a wage-price freeze and the Economic Stabilization Program (ESP) by proposing stringent limits on Medicare reimbursement. The Cost of Living Council (CLC) rejected their proposals as beyond ESP authority, which the Council defined as restricted to limits on aggregate hospital revenue. A CLC staff member described BHI's proposal as "a classic case of bureaucracy doing under somebody else's authority what they couldn't do under their own law." SSA withdrew, remaining involved in ESP regulations only to ensure that ongoing arrangements with providers would not be disrupted.[P]

Within the Medicare program, BHI officials demonstrated a similar predilection for ceilings on reimbursement. Although their superiors in SSA and HEW proposed prospective reimbursement, which could theoretically entail financial rewards as well as reimbursement limits, BHI officials favored the latter. They had proposed their consideration internally even before prospective reimbursement became politically popular but met with immediate resistance. Thus they were pleased when the staff of the Ways and Means Committee supported their approach by proposing to authorize ceilings on reimbursement, while restricting general prospective reimbursement authority to experimentation.[28]

BHI scepticism toward financial incentives and reimbursement experimentation, along with their preference for the establishment of ceilings, derived from their experience with reimbursement and their desire to achieve control over excesses. Experience had taught them that all institutions would try to get as much money as they could from the government and would hold onto any payment advantages they were granted. The result was loss of control over program expenditures. The only way officials saw to regain control in this situation was to avoid opening the door to new demands, creating new loopholes, and allowing any further financial exploitation of the Medicare trust fund. This attitude explains not only their scepticism toward experimentation and prospective reimbursement, but also their advocacy of restricting the certification

---

[P]Discussed in detail in *Character and Implications,* Chapter VI. It is based on interviews with participating BHI and CLC officials.

of the renal-dialysis facilities,[q] and their persistent opposition to capitation reimbursement for prepaid group practices or, later, HMOs. As a counter to the Nixon administration's market approach to HMO development, Irwin Wolkstein of BHI proposed a narrow, carefully monitored demonstration.

> . . . it is not feasible to select, monitor and evaluate a large number—100 or more—highly experimental situations; the level of personnel involved in evaluating potential HMOs will necessarily be not very highly skilled if the workload is large; once you approve an approach because it has turned out badly the chances of getting rid of it are very poor—vested interests develop.[29]

Although advocates of rapid and widespread HMO development argued that any problems of this sort would work themselves out through competition, BHI officials feared the trust fund would go bankrupt in the process.[30] To ward off new demands on Medicare funds, BHI officials opposed any measure that would cost the program more money, regardless of the savings it might achieve for the health-care system as a whole. As they subordinated innovation to efforts to prevent waste, existing reimbursement policy became further entrenched in spite of its recognized problems and inadequacies.

The defensiveness apparent in BHI's attitude on cost control characterizes SSA's general response to growing Congressional and Executive efforts to influence Medicare policy. Most active within Congress has been the Senate Finance Committee. Although staff of that committee have frequently supported BHI objectives in pursuit of their own interests on Medicare oversight, they have challenged SSA independence. SSA opposed the development of Professional Standards Review Organizations (PSROs) largely for this reason.[r]

The handling of PSROs also reveals the threat within HEW to SSA's control over the Medicare program. As Medicare's size has dwarfed all other health programs, the Secretary of HEW and Assistant Secretary for Health have increased their efforts to assert control over the independent SSA.[31] Because HEW was more responsive to Senator Bennett's PSRO proposal, the Finance Committee delegated authority for its implementation to the Assistant Secretary rather than to SSA.[32] The Secretary has also required that SSA share authority over several other recently legislated provisions of the Medicare law. In addition, the Office of Management and Budget, sometimes with HEW support, has forced SSA to develop regulations inconsistent with the latter's political objectives. Notable in this respect are the withdrawal of current financing and proposed

---

[q]Discussed briefly in *Character and Implications*, Chapter VII. It is based on interviews with BHI officials; "Final Policies PL 92-603, Section 2991, "End-Stage Renal Disease Program of Medicare," 1974, Office of Policy Development and Planning, Office of the Assistant Secretary for Health, HEW, Office of the Secretary, Washington, D.C.

[r]Discussed in *Character and Implications,* Chapter V. It is based on interviews with BHI and congressional officials.

changes in utilization review. In both cases, SSA opposed proposal of the regulations as creating more controversy than they were worth, but they were overruled.[s]

Increasingly, SSA's authority over their program has been undermined. Although partially a product of the suspicion and distrust of the Nixon years, the basic issue is who is responsible for the major health-policy decisions entailed in administering Medicare. Because increased executive authority over SSA would reduce congressional influence on its activity, there has been support in Congress, particularly in the tax committees, for SSA's continued responsibility and independence. But the agency's status remains unresolved, and SSA is politically weaker now than it was when Medicare was enacted. As its Medicare problems are compounded by the deficits appearing in its old age, survivors, and disability trust funds, SSA is increasingly on the defensive.

Implications for Future Policy

Identifying the bureaucratic characteristics that have shaped SSA's administration of Medicare is useful not only for understanding that program but also for suggesting what to expect from an SSA role in any extension of federal health insurance. These expectations depend on the kind of role SSA is given. Specifically, the impact on policy of SSA's predominant characteristics will vary with two major determinants of its political environment: (1) the portion of the nation's health care for which SSA becomes fiscally responsible, and the terms of that responsibility; and (2) the degree to which SSA has sole administrative authority or shares it with others. The matrix shown in table 2-1 indicates the alternatives SSA's position could take. Theoretically, it is possible to fill all the cells in this matrix, but this discussion will focus on the alternatives most relevant to deliberations on expanding federal health insurance.

Alternative 1 would have SSA—independent of HEW—responsible for financing all health services, with total expenditures prescribed in the executive budget. This arrangement obviously bears a marked resemblance to Senator Kennedy's labor-supported Health Security Act. In theory, including all health-care costs in the federal budget, putting a ceiling upon them, and giving full responsibility for them to a single government agency maximizes government's incentives to control health-care costs effectively and rationally.[33] SSA's behavior under Medicare illustrates that political attention to federal expenditures and administrators' desires to keep their program under control lead to efforts to control costs. But as long as government responsibility is limited to a segment of health-care costs, administrators focus on the costs of their program, not on

---

[s]Discussed in *Character and Implications,* Chapter VII. It is based on interviews with BHI officials.

Table 2-1
Alternative SSA Program Goals

Fiscal Responsibility for and Comprehensiveness of Health-Insurance Coverage	Federally Funded Comprehensive Coverage for all Citizens, with Ceilings on Expenditures	Federally Funded Comprehensive Coverage for all Citizens, with No Ceilings on Expenditures	Federally Funded Coverage for Groups or Specific Health-Care Costs	Privately Financed, Federally Mandated Coverage for All or Some Health-Care Costs
Administrative Authority				
Authority in a single federal agency	1.	2.		
Authority divided among federal agencies		3.	4.	
Authority divided between state and federal governments			5.	
Authority divided between the federal government and private insurers				6.

health care as a whole. Consequently, as Medicare illustrates, rational action for the overall system is rejected if it impinges negatively on the program in question. Centralizing expenditures and administrative responsibility, making program costs identical to total costs, theoretically gets around this problem.

In practice, however, this arrangement demands a totally different kind of political and administrative approach than SSA has demonstrated under Medicare, and, consequently, would considerably strain the bureaucracy. Full fiscal responsibility for all health-care costs would increase several-fold the pressures under which SSA has been operating. Totally dependent on the government for all their revenue, hospitals could be expected to exercise their full political muscle against SSA in establishing terms for payment and overall surveillance. Within the Executive, SSA could expect similar pressure from the President and other departments, all of whom would perceive health-care expenditures as a threat to their own needs for funds.[34] Having to establish an overall health budget, and budgets for regions and hospitals all down the line, would thus place SSA in an adversary position vis-a-vis both the industry and other government agencies.

Over the past ten years SSA has diligently tried not to appear as an industry adversary, continuously avoiding controversy by keeping its bargains and maintaining established procedures. Its efforts to compromise competing interests and achieve political consensus have not entirely worked, as evidenced by recent criticism of the agency. As a result, SSA has become increasingly defensive with respect to Executive and Congressional efforts to influence program operations. Were SSA to be delegated the above responsibility for national health insurance, the contradiction between its task and its experience and political strategy would become so great as to seriously undermine its capacity to act.

Much of this analysis would also apply to adoption of alternatives 2 or 3, most clearly resembling the 1974 Kennedy-Mills bill. A key difference between these and the first alternative is the reduction in pressure that follows from eliminating responsibility for budget setting. Without the requirement for budgets and ceilings, confronting rising costs remains the political matter it has been in the past, and SSA's task would be more like its present one than would be above. Accordingly, along with an increase in administrative stress, we would expect persistence of the agency's present approach to policy and policy making. Officials would avoid change wherever possible and, when forced to exercise control over the industry, would opt for the least controversial methods. As we have seen, this approach leads to reluctance to innovate in the payment area and avoidance of quality enforcement.

The third column of the matrix presents arrangements that would apply to extensions of Medicare like catastrophic coverage, coverage of the unemployed, children, and so on, and federalizing Medicaid. In terms of policy deliberations, these seem most appropriately placed in cell 4. The consequences of such extensions for SSA's performance would vary with their cost and the nature of the covered group. Any extension of coverage adds to provider pressure on SSA as it increases the proportion of health costs and provider revenues paid for by government. The larger the share of costs, the greater the pressure. None of the above extensions, however, seems likely to overwhelm SSA, leaving the agency to handle them just as they have administered Medicare. We would expect SSA to focus on getting the program operating smoothly and to avoid interference in the health-care industry, with cost-control measures restricted as in the past to program costs rather than health-care costs in general. SSA willingness to shift cost burdens to beneficiaries through limited payment or reliance on patient cost sharing is likely to vary with the political power associated with the group covered. Thus, for example, if SSA covered the poor, they would seem more likely to limit reimbursement than if they covered children. This would also apply if SSA became responsible for Medicaid administration under the present federal-state format (alternative 5). On the other hand, encompassing the poor in the same program with groups better able to protect themselves, like the elderly, might in fact protect the weak groups. Thus the implications are somewhat unclear, but policy seems likely to be influenced by the direction of SSA expansion—toward the poor or middle classes.

A very different approach to expanding federal health insurance is represented by alternative 6. In this category falls the privately financed, mandated approach to expanding health-insurance coverage, whether for the whole population or a segment of it. If federal supervision of mandated health insurance were delegated to the Social Security Administration or, as is more likely, if SSA continued to be responsible for certain segments of the population not covered by private insurance, certain policy implications would follow. If charged with developing and enforcing overall or simply payment regulations for mandated coverage by private health insurance, SSA would have little incentive to impose restrictions on the insurance or health-care industries. Blame for poor performance would most likely be laid at the insurance industry's doorstep, rather than the executive agency's, and costs would not appear in the executive budget. Thus, even if SSA promulgated relatively restrictive regulations, they would be unlikely to stringently enforce them. Extending this analysis to any direct fiscal responsibility SSA would retain (e.g., Medicare) or acquire, SSA would be in a position to impose limits on its own reimbursement, leaving the private sector to pick up the tab in hospital expenditures. The escape valve of private payment would reduce provider pressure on SSA, and the absence of centralized fiscal responsibility would inhibit effective overall cost control.

These predictions as to what to expect from SSA in the future are based on the agency's characteristics in 1975, after ten years of Medicare experience. Their usefulness does not rest on the assumption that agencies cannot change; they can. But if policy is to achieve the results its designers intend, policy makers must take into account the existing tendencies and biases that will shape implementation. In so doing, they can develop legislation that will more effectively serve the purpose for which it is enacted.

3

Implementation of the End-Stage Renal-Disease Program: A Mixed Pattern of Subsidizing and Regulating the Delivery of Medical Services

Richard A. Rettig and
Thomas C. Webster

End-stage renal[a] disease is that clinical condition reached when an individual has experienced such a degree of irreversible deterioration of kidney function that—without treatment—death will soon follow. The two principal means of treating end-stage renal disease are *hemodialysis*, cleansing the metabolic waste products in the blood by use of the artificial-kidney machine, and renal transplantation.

The costs of dialysis have always been high. Based upon 1972 data for 10 home-dialysis programs in 6 states and 96 center-dialysis programs (81 hospital and 15 nonhospital) in 11 states and 2 counties, a recent General Accounting Office (GAO)[1] study indicated charges approaching $50,000 per patient. (See Table 3-1.)

Table 3-1
Annual Cost of Dialysis

	Center Dialysis			Home Dialysis	
	Total (96)	Hospital (81)	Nonhospital (15)	1st Year	2nd Year
Average Charge	$30,100	$30,500	$27,600	$14,900	$7,000
Range		11,500–49,100	12,800–46,800		

Source: Comptroller General of the United States, "Treatment of Chronic Kidney Failure: Dialysis, Transplant, Costs and the Need For More Vigorous Efforts" (Washington, D.C.: U.S. General Accounting Office, June 24, 1975), pp. 38–39.
Note: Data are for 1972.

The costs of transplantation are also significant. Charges during 1973 in 24 facilities analyzed by the GAO ranged from $5,500 to $20,500 and averaged about $12,800. The Department of Health, Education, and Welfare (HEW) cited costs to the GAO of $14,000 for a living related donor transplant. Included in

This chapter is part of a larger research project: "Kidney Therapy and Public Policy," supported by National Science Foundation Grant No. GI-39327 and begun while the authors were at the Ohio State University. Results of the work on the larger project will be available in 1977.

[a]*Renal* means pertaining to the kidneys, from *ren*, the Latin word for kidney.

the costs were hospital room, board, ancillary charges, and professional fees.[2]

The costs of therapy to a given individual can vary substantially according to the therapy or combination of therapies received and a number of other contingencies. The general point, however, is that neither type of therapy is inexpensive, although for the individual patient a successful transplant is by far the least costly.

The number of beneficiaries of end-stage renal disease treatment is fairly small relative to the population. The number of reported dialysis patients alive in July 1970, 1971, and 1972 was 2,874, 4,375, and 5,786, respectively.[b] The total number of kidney transplants reported for 1967, 1968, 1969, 1970, and 1971, respectively, was 428, 625, 787, 996, and 1,172.[c]

In Public Law 92-603, the Social Security Amendments of 1972, Medicare health-insurance coverage for end-stage renal disease was effectively extended to more than 90 percent of the United States population. The 1965 law, which established Medicare, provided health-insurance coverage to the aged—those over 65 years of age, and this included coverage for renal failure.[3] Restrictive patient selection criteria for hemodialysis and renal-transplantation patients, and limited knowledge of this specific form of the general benefit, however, resulted in relatively few individuals receiving Medicare benefits for end-stage renal disease before 1973.

Public Law 92-603, enacted on October 30, 1972, provided Medicare coverage to the under-65 population in two ways. First, those individuals under age 65 who qualified for cash benefits under social security or the railroad-retirement system because of a *disability* so incapacitating that they were prevented from working became eligible, after a 24-month waiting period, for Medicare's hospital and supplementary medical-insurance protection.[4] This protection included coverage for end-stage renal disease.

A substantial number of potential end-stage renal-disease patients, approximately 60 percent of the total, however, could not qualify for Medicare

---

[b]See Research Triangle Institute, *The National Dialysis Registry: Second Annual Progress Report, July 1, 1969 – June 30, 1970*, August 1970; *Third Annual Progress Report, July 1, 1970 – June 30, 1971*, July 1971; and *Fourth Annual Progress Report, July 1, 1971 – June 30, 1972*, July 1972. The national dialysis-patient load reported in January 1971, January 1972, January 1973, and January 1974, respectively, was 16.6 cases per million population, 24.4 per million, 37.4 per million, and 46.9 per million. See National Institutes of Health, *Proceedings of the 4th, 5th, 6th, and 7th Annual Contractors Conference of the Artificial Kidney Program of the National Institute of Arthritis and Metabolic Diseases*, Washington, D.C., 1971, 1972, 1973, and 1974.

[c]See National Institutes of Health, *U.S. Kidney Transplant Fact Book: Information from ACS/NIH Registry, 1972*, Washington, D.C., 1972. There are several indications that data supplied to the American College of Surgeons/National Institutes of Health Organ Transplant Registry underreport the kidney transplants performed in the United States by nearly 50 percent. For an analysis of this problem see Sr. Josephine Sullivan, "The Role of Data In End-Stage Renal Disease Programs," M.S. Thesis, Hospital and Health Services Administration, Ohio State University, 1975.

on either the basis of age or entitlement to cash disability benefits. Medicare coverage was extended to this larger group by Sec. 2991 of the act. Sec. 2991 stipulated that every individual not yet 65 years old, who was fully or currently insured or entitled to monthly insurance benefits under social security, or who was the spouse or dependent child of such an individual, and who was "medically determined to have chronic renal disease" and to require hemodialysis or renal transplantation, shall, in the language of the act, "be deemed to be disabled for purposes of coverage under parts A and B of Medicare subject to the deductible, premium, and copayment provisions of Title XVIII."[5]

The End-Stage Renal Disease Program (ESRD) as established by Public Law 92-603 was primarily intended to subsidize the costs of providing therapy. The provision of a subsidy, however, was accompanied by regulatory constraints. The language of the statute required that the Secretary of Health, Education, and Welfare establish minimum utilization rates and medical review boards. Both of these requirements were intended to regulate the quality of care. Although it was not mentioned in the statute, cost control was also a regulatory objective.

The emergence of cost control as an objective of regulation is attributable to several factors. The entire 1972 legislation was permeated with a desire to control the costs of Medicare, which had continuously escalated since its enactment in 1965. Since the ESRD program established nearly universal coverage for kidney failure, the private market was essentially eliminated as a basis for determining the "reasonable cost" and "reasonable charge" of treatment.[d] An alternative to standard Medicare procedures had to be developed for reimbursement purposes. Consequently, as HEW officials articulated the ESRD program's goals, they included cost control as a major objective.

Cost control remains a continuing concern of policy makers for the ESRD program. The program, which went into effect on July 1, 1973, estimated incurred costs for the first year at $150 million for Sec. 2991 beneficiaries and an additional $100 million for patients eligible under the aged and disabled provisions. The estimated incurred costs for the first, second, third, and fourth years for both Sec. 2991 and all Medicare renal patients are shown in table 3-2.[6] It is estimated that the annual costs for renal-disease patients will exceed $1 billion by 1984.

The number of renal-disease patients who had qualified for Medicare coverage as of March 31, 1975, under all three provisions, was 25,066, of whom

---

[d]For a discussion of Medicare reimbursement principles and procedures, see Herman M. Somers and Anne R. Somers, *Medicare and the Hospitals: Issues and Prospects,* Washington, D.C., Brookings Institution, 1967, pp. 154-196; Robert J. Myers, *Medicare,* Homewood, Illinois, Richard D. Irwin, Inc., 1970, pp. 128-153; U.S. Senate, Committee on Finance, *Medicare and Medicaid: Problems, Issues, and Alternatives,* Staff Report, 91st Congress, 2nd Session, 1970, pp. 45-89; and Sylvia A. Law, *Blue Cross: What Went Wrong?,* New Haven, Yale University Press, 1974, pp. 59-102.

Table 3-2
Estimated Medicare-Incurred Costs of End-Stage Renal
Disease (*in millions*)

	Fiscal Year			
	1974	1975	1976	1977
Sec. 299I patients	$150	$225	$300	$360
All renal patients	$250	$350	$500	$600

Source: U.S. House of Representatives, Committee on Ways and
Means, "Background Information on Kidney Disease Benefits Under
Medicare," Committee Print, 94th Congress, 1st Session, June 24,
1975, p. 3.

20,764 were living.[7] 60 percent of the total was qualified on the basis of Sec.
299I. Estimates are that the number of patients alive and receiving renal-disease
benefits will rise by 50,000 to 70,000 by 1990. The magnitude of the resource
requirements for the small number of beneficiaries, then, is a constant stimulus
to cost control.

It is important to emphasize that cost control within the ESRD program is
a secondary objective. The ESRD program's primary purpose is to subsidize the
provision of medical services. We have, therefore, another instance of the mixed
pattern of subsidy and regulation as the means for achieving public-policy
objectives.[e]

Within this context of subsidy and regulation, the ESRD program stands out
as a potential prototype of either a catastrophic health-insurance program or a
more comprehensive national health-insurance program. End-stage renal disease
was not thought to be a typical disease, but the ESRD program was and is
thought to constitute a small-scale "experiment" to test the administrative
capability of the federal government to handle national health insurance.[f]

The purpose of this chapter is to analyze the cost-control strategy of the
Social Security Administration and the Department of Health, Education, and
Welfare in the design and execution of the ESRD Interim Program. From this

[e]See Allen V. Kneese and Charles L. Schultze, *Pollution, Prices, and Public Policy,* Washington, D.C., Brookings, 1975, for a critical discussion on the use of subsidy and regulation
to achieve water quality and an argument for the substitution of an incentive system including effluent charges. Providing ESRD medical services and controlling water quality
are asymmetric, of course; one is directed to encouraging the private sector to produce
an economic good and the other is intended to dissuade the private sector from producing
an economic "bad."

[f]In B.D. Cohen, "Treatment Program Cost Questioned," *Washington Post,* June 17, 1975,
Senator Russell B. Long, chairman of the Senate Finance Committee, was quoted as saying:
"It's a forerunner [for catastrophic-health insurance] and will definitely give us a lot of
help in deciding how it can be administered."

analysis we attempt to draw some lessons for any future program of national health insurance.

The ESRD Interim Program

Origins

Public Law 92-603 stipulated that the end-stage renal disease provision was to become effective on July 1, 1973. It was not until June 29, however, just three days before this date, that interim regulations were published in the *Federal Register.*[8] These implementing regulations deal primarily with reimbursement issues and not at all with the two quality-of-care requirements of the law— minimum utilization rates and medical review boards. At this writing, the ESRD program is still being administered under these interim regulations.[g]

The decision to separate reimbursement from quality-of-care issues and to deal with the former in an interim program arose from two sources. First, renal disease was a new and practically unknown phenomenon for the Social Security Administration's (SSA) Bureau of Health Insurance (BHI). Although Medicare had provided end-stage renal-disease benefits for those over 65 prior to July 1, 1973, the beneficiaries were few and the administrative experience was not especially informative for administering the new program. Moreover, Sec. 2991 was an unanticipated part of the 1972 legislation.[h] In the prolonged legislative history of H.R. 1, which became P.L. 92-603, no hearings were held in either the House or the Senate on end-stage renal disease,[i] and Sec. 2991 was

---

[g]On July 1, 1975, fully two years later, proposed final regulations were published; see "Conditions for Coverage of Suppliers of End-Stage Renal Disease (ESRD) Services," *Federal Register*, Vol. 40, No. 127, July 1, 1975, pp. 27782–27793. A 60-day period was provided for public comments. Consideration of these comments will occur before final adoption of the proposed regulations. The publication, therefore, of "final" final regulations might be expected in late 1975 or early 1976. On most of the major issues in the proposed final regulations, however, implementation has already been initiated.

[h]It is true that the Gottschalk Committee Report, in 1967, had recommended patient-care financing for ESRD through Title XVIII of the Social Security Act. That recommendation was then incorporated into a number of legislative proposals, but nothing came of this approach until 1972. See *Report of the Committee on Chronic Kidney Disease,* Washington, D.C., September 1967, p. 14.

[i]The House Ways and Means Committee did receive testimony by dialysis patients on November 4, 1971, and from William J. Flanigan, M.D., on November 11, but this was in connection with national health insurance, not with H.R. 1 to which the ESRD provision would later be attached. See U.S. House of Representatives, Committee on Ways Representatives, Committee on Ways and Means, *National Health Insurance Proposals,* Hearings, Pt. 7, pp. 1524–1546, and Pt. 10, pp. 2226–2228, 92nd Congress, 1st Session, 1971. Subsequent to these hearings, Rep. Wilbur Mills introduced a bill to provide financing for patients with end-stage renal disease, but this also was never the subject of hearings.

incorporated into the bill on the Senate floor just one month before the act was signed into law.[9] In response to this new provision, BHI established a task force on chronic kidney disease immediately upon enactment of the law in order to educate itself on the requirements for implementing the ESRD program. The task force and higher level BHI officials soon discovered that the treatment of end-stage renal disease was highly complex.

BHI further discovered in the degree of administrative complexity within HEW the second source of the interim program. Administrative complexity arose mainly from ambiguity about how the HEW Secretary's authority would be exercised in the ESRD program. Since the ESRD program was part of Medicare, it might be expected that responsibility for its implementation would be delegated to the Commissioner of Social Security and by him to the BHI. Since the Commissioner reports directly to the Secretary, it might further be expected that BHI would have substantial autonomy in the administration of the ESRD program.

The Assistant Secretary for Health of HEW, although lacking line authority over the Social Security Commissioner, had recently been given the responsibility for coordinating Medicare issues with the other health concerns of HEW. The manner in which this coordination was to occur, however, was not an established administrative procedure.[j] The role of "H", as the health activity of HEW is bureaucratically known, was carved out by the forceful insertion of Dr. Ronald Klar, on behalf of the Assistant Secretary, into the regulation writing process. Klar's efforts brought about a sharing of responsibility between SSA and "H", although the resulting conflict threatened serious delay in issuing the implementing regulations.[k] The technical complexity of treating end-stage

---

[j]The administrative complexity was even greater than indicated in the text, although this chapter is not the vehicle for fully explicating this dimension. The Kidney Disease Control Program (KDCP), which had existed since 1965, was the principal source of bureaucratic competence within the federal government at the time of passage of P.L. 92-603. The BHI task force began asking the KDCP for assistance in November 1972, which the latter cooperatively provided. The fate of the KDCP was sealed in early 1973, however, when the Nixon administration's budget request to the Congress for fiscal 1974 contained no funds for the Regional Medical Program Service, of which the KDCP was a part. In its waning months, the KDCP not only provided assistance and information to BHI, but also provided staff support for Klar as he involved himself in the regulation writing process. Furthermore, although KDCP expired by the end of the fiscal year, "H" reconstituted an end-stage renal-disease unit, this time within the Bureau of Quality Assurance (BQA), by August 1973. The End-Stage Renal Disease Division of BQA has had relatively little to do with the design of the interim program and only somewhat more to do with its execution; it has been primarily engaged in design of the long-range program. Parenthetically, this episode highlights the prospective problem of effectively using existing sources of competence in "health" when national health insurance becomes a reality.

[k]We again note parenthetically a general problem that prospectively confronts the nation in any national health-insurance program, namely, the resolution of respective authorities and responsibilities of the Office of the Secretary of Health, Education, and Welfare and those of the Commissioner of the Social Security Administration.

renal disease, the administrative complexity of relations between SSA and "H", and the necessity of issuing implementing regulations resulted in the decision to issue interim regulations, which covered the essential reimbursement issues, and to leave the more complicated organizational questions to be resolved later. These interim regulations were published in the late spring of 1973.

The Implementation-Issue Structure

The implementation of public policy can be understood as a process of transforming public policy objectives into policy outputs that approximate the initial policy intentions. In fact, there are numerous multidimensional transformations that occur as policy is implemented.

One important transformation is the conversion of policy objectives from ends-oriented statements to means-oriented statements. We refer to this as the transformation of the goal structure into the implementation-issue structure. The implementation-issue structure represents a factoring of the goal structure into administrative processes and subprocesses, and constitutes a map to sources of potential conflict. This instrumental factoring of goals into administrative processes is especially important because it establishes the frame of reference within which both the design and execution of program implementation occurs.

The administrative processes into which the policy goals and objectives are factored will depend, of course, on the bureaucratic situation existing at the outset of the implementation process. If an established organization will administer the policy, the implementation issue structure will be determined mainly by preexisting, standard operating procedures.[1] If a new organization is to administer the policy, the implementation-issue structure will become a template used to design new procedures.

The goal structure of the ESRD program included the following:[10]

1. The guarantee of access to ESRD medical services by all those eligible for such care
2. The provision of high-quality care
3. The assurance of efficient and economical allocation and use of medical resources
4. The containment of costs

Since the interim program for end-stage renal disease addressed itself mainly to the urgent issues of reimbursement, the primary administrative responsibility

---

[1] See Graham T. Allison, *Essence of Decision: Explaining the Cuban Missile Crisis*, Boston, Little, Brown and Company, 1971, esp. pp. 67–100, for a discussion of the importance of standard operating procedures, programs, and repertoires in organizational behavior.

for implementation fell to the BHI. Not surprisingly, therefore, the implementation-issue structure was derived from standard Medicare categories. Included were the following six items:

1. Patient eligibility
2. Patient entitlement
3. Facility certification
4. Covered services
5. Facility reimbursement
6. Physician reimbursement

The first two of these issues—patient eligibility and entitlement—were spelled out in all essential details in the law, with some further elaboration in the interim regulations. These issues, although critical to program implementation, do not bear directly on the cost-control efforts of the ESRD program. The latter four issues, however, constitute the heart of the cost-control strategy for this program.

The Cost-Control Strategy

Facility Certification. The program planners wanted to initiate the ESRD program in a way that restricted sudden growth in the number of provider facilities on the eve of the establishment of a guaranteed patient market. A "freeze" was placed on new facilities in an effort to maintain or increase the utilization rates for the covered procedures until the minimum utilization rates could be developed for the long-range program, or until procedures for permitting treatment capacity to grow in relation to increased patient demand could be developed.[11] The interim regulations, therefore, limited certification in general to facilities that were providing end-stage renal-disease treatment prior to June 1, 1973, and that had not substantially increased their services at the time of the regulations. Transplant hospitals, which had been participating in the Medicare program, would continue to be reimbursed in the interim period for renal transplantation until further conditions of participation were promulgated and applied.

Dialysis facilities that met the above general conditions would be certified if they met the following "minimal conditions":

(1) If hospital operated, the hospital is participating in the Medicare program; (2) if free-standing, the facility (a) meets State or local licensure requirements, if any, (b) is a facility in which treatment is under the general supervision of a physician (who need not be a full-time supervisor), (c) has an affiliation, e.g., has arrangements for back-up care, etc., with a participating hospital, and (d) agrees that no charge will be made for a covered dialysis service provided by the facility that is in excess of the charge determined to be the reasonable charge of that facility.[12]

Based upon information about transplantation and dialysis facilities provided by the Comprehensive Health Planning (CHP) Program and the Regional Medical Program Service of HEW at the request of the BHI, a list of certified facilities was compiled by the SSA in early 1973. The initial design decision about facility certification, therefore, was to "grandfather" in all those facilities providing services on the eve of the program's becoming operational and to impose a freeze on expansion of their services and creation of new facilities.

At the same time that the freeze on new facilities and the expansion of existing ones was being imposed, policy makers recognized that additional treatment capacity would be needed to handle increased patient demand. So, in August 1973, the task of developing "exception criteria and procedures" for the certification of new facilities and the disposition of requests by existing facilities to expand was given to the newly created End-Stage Renal Disease Program in the Bureau of Quality Assurance (BQA/ESRD) of HEW. This task was deemed to be "medical" and not "financial" and therefore was allocated to the "H" side of HEW. The process of drafting the criteria and procedures statement, informally clearing the statement with the field, and securing higher level bureaucratic clearance took four months, but approval came for the statement's release in early December.[13]

There then began the adjudication process by which applications for permission to build new facilities or expand existing ones were submitted to the government and processed. A quite lengthy chain of review, beginning with the initial submission of an application to a local CHP "B" agency, eventually would lead to a five-member adjudication group in HEW. This group, composed of two individuals from the BHI, two from the BQA/ESRD unit, and one from the CHP program, reviews applications and recommends that they be approved, deferred pending submission of more information, or disapproved. These recommendations are then transmitted to the SSA for final disposition.

In general, the adjudication group has been very reluctant to approve any additional transplantation capacity on the grounds that sufficient capacity currently exists. Criteria for approving new dialysis facilities have included (1) an assessment of need based upon the number of patients requiring care and the capacity of other dialysis facilities in a given geographic area and (2) consideration of the estimated maximum time a patient would have to travel in order to reach a dialysis facility.

Close observers of the adjudication process have indicated that SSA has been reluctant to disapprove an application, even when disapproval has been recommended by the adjudication work group. In this certification process, substantial rights are given to facilities providing treatment, and a disapproved application can easily become a litigated court case. Since the SSA must represent the United States government in court if a disapproved application is litigated, the legal advice it is given strongly recommends accepting for litigation only those cases the government is likely to win. In the close case, therefore, the benefit of the doubt is given to the applying facility.

The certification of facilities is seen by HEW as a way to avoid undue build-up of capacity and to ensure adequate use of existing facilities. In essence, the certification process is a cost-control process. Generally, this process has been employed to permit capacity to increase in accordance with increasing patient demand. But one cannot overlook the BHI's hesitancy to disapprove facility certification applications. The establishment of bureaucratic mechanisms for implementing cost-control incentives in the ESRD program is significantly affected by the threat of litigation. Prospectively, any national health-insurance program will also confront this same problem.

Covered Services. A major problem in third-party financing of health services, as Sylvester Berki[14] has noted, is that the nature of the health product is seldom specified. Without such specification there is no enforceable limit on the quantity or quality of health services provided. Although the requirement that there be a local medical review board held out the promise of a process by which medically unnecessary services would be limited, that requirement remains to be implemented. In the absence of the review board, the interim program sought to eliminate the unnecessary services in two major areas with great potential for abuse—the extent of use of laboratory procedures and the provision of physician services for stabilized patients.

The implementing instrument in each case, however, was not the published interim regulations but the initial intermediary letter issued by the SSA.[15] The intermediary letter listed those laboratory procedures that could be employed and the frequency with which they could be employed without additional medical justification. Additional tests beyond those on the list, or tests at a greater frequency than indicated, had to be accompanied by a statement of medical necessity if the provider was to be reimbursed.

In a similar manner, office visits for stabilized patients were limited to one per month and extensive examinations to two per year. This restriction, however, quickly became one of the most controversial in the actual implementation of the new program, although not as controversial as the issue of physician reimbursement. It was thought to reflect the clinical views of the Seattle dialyzers and clearly did not reflect consensus among clinicians regarding standard medical practice.

Although these restrictions on physician services came under sharp attack, they were not modified. But the difficulty in proscribing such services was spelled out in December 1973 in a memorandum to the Assistant Secretary for Health from the director of the Office of Health Financing Policy Development:

While it is . . . appropriate to reimburse for these [routine physician] services, it would seem reasonable to expect that some standards of "acceptable" medical practice could be established for these services. Development of criteria has been most difficult for the category of routine physician services during maintenance dialysis. The kinds and amount of "supervision" have varied considerably by physician and area as well as by patient, ranging from "on-call" availability to performing routine physical examinations. Consultations with numerous professionals have failed to yield a consensus on professional standards--we cannot specify or quantify any one set of services constituting acceptable medical practice.[16]

The regulation of covered services, the ESRD program's experience would suggest, depends upon there being an ascertainable and respected point of view within the physician community regarding standard medical practice. That point of view need not reflect widespread consensus within the physician community. On the other hand, given the discrepancies that exist in the provision of ESRD program's services, it may not be possible to establish widespread consensus. The absence of widespread consensus, however, suggests there are substantial difficulties in imposing the "best" medical practice as the norm for all physicians.

Facility Reimbursement. In a departure from prior Medicare practice, the interim regulations indicated that "customary and prevailing charges" could not be used as a basis for reimbursing facilities providing end-stage renal-disease services.[17] The reason for this was quite simple. The nearly universal coverage established for ESRD by Sec. 2991 effectively eliminated the normal medical market as a basis for establishing reimbursement rates. Instead, the regulations called for reasonable charges for services defined in relation to "charges or costs prior to July 1, 1973, [to] the costs and profits that are reasonable when the treatments are provided in an effective and economical manner, and/or [to the] charges made for other services, taking into account comparable physicians' time and skill requirements."[18]

The implementing intermediary letter indicated that screens of $150 per dialysis for maintenance dialysis and $190 for self-dialysis training would constitute the basis for reasonable charges.[19] Although the BHI emphasized that a screen was not a ceiling, all charges above these levels had to be justified before they would be reimbursed. The screens, therefore, effectively functioned as ceilings on reimbursable charges for participating facilities.

From a cost-control standpoint, the screen for maintenance dialysis was designed to provide an incentive toward efficiency for those facilities whose costs were higher than $150 per dialysis. However, no incentives toward efficiency were provided to facilities able to deliver dialysis at less than the $150 level. Some physicians reacted to this latter fact by suggesting that the government permit facilities billing below the screens to capture a portion of the savings for their own purposes. No action was taken on this suggestion, however, and charges by the more efficient providers have moved upward toward the screen.

It was the widely shared intention among policy makers in Congress, the Office of the HEW Secretary, and BHI to create cost-containment incentives in the implementation of the ESRD program. It is also important to note that there were strong voices within the nephrology community urging the government to take effective action in limiting total program costs through the establishment of incentives for cost control. Government policy on limiting facility reimbursement, in short, had substantial support among a significant portion of the specialist medical community.

Two factors have been at work to modify the initial screens. First, there has been a steady differentiation of dialysis treatments and a corollary differentiation of appropriate screens. In July 1974, for example, the $150 to $190 screens were removed on inpatient-dialysis services and reimbursement was to be based instead upon "a reasonable cost basis in the same manner as any other inpatient services *when the inpatient stay is determined to be reasonable and medically necessary*."[20] The second factor affecting the screens has been the form of physician reimbursement to which we turn next.

The costs of providing ESRD services, of course, are vulnerable to the effects of inflation. Although no adjustment has yet been made for inflation, one will probably occur in the near future in accordance with standard Medicare procedures. In any event, the most effective means of cost containment that has been employed in the implementation of the ESRD program has been the use of the screens on facility reimbursement for dialysis services.

Physician Reimbursement. One of the most startling features of the intermediary letter, which followed the interim regulations, was the requirement that physicians be paid out of the reimbursement to the facility.[m] Not surprisingly, this departure from fee-for-service billing procedures aroused a storm of protest from the medical community.

This protest was by no means a unanimous expression of opinion among nephrologists engaged in the clinical practice of dialysis. Many such individuals had been among the pioneers in providing dialysis services to patients prior to the 1972 legislation under circumstances where boot-strap economy was the prevailing practice. These economizing pioneers frequently had an academic affiliation or were institutionally based without a private practice and thus constituted a salaried physician group. This group, in many ways, was extremely

---

[m]U.S. Department of Health, Education, and Welfare, Social Security Administration, Part A Intermediary Letter No. 73-25, Part B Intermediary Letter No. 73-22, "Processing and Payment of Claims for Renal Dialysis and Transplant Services Performed for Eligible Medicare Beneficiaries after June 30, 1973," July 1973, pp. 16–17; "Furthermore, with respect to physicians' services, for each routine dialysis performed there will be recognized only a facility component of service; consequently, the cost of the administrative and supervisory role of the physician in the facility would be recognized only as part of the facility overhead, and included in the renal dialysis cost center."

influential at the outset of the ESRD program in urging cost-containment incentives upon the government.

But this group hardly spoke for all nephrologists. There were also a substantial number of nephrologists in private practice, usually in situations where third-party financing had been established, who had discovered that quite a good living could be made by dialyzing patients. In fact, there developed several proprietary dialysis-providing enterprises, at least one of which was nationwide in scope.[n] To be made salaried employees of the facilities in which they dialyzed patients was outrageous to many of these nephrologists.

This is not the place to record in full the protest over physician reimbursement, but a brief overview is appropriate. Perhaps auspiciously, the protest began on Friday, July 13, 1973, at a hotel near Chicago's O'Hare Airport where sixty or more nephrologists from across the country met to express their strong concern about the elimination of fee-for-service reimbursement. One result of that meeting was the establishment of the Physicians for Renal Replacement Therapy, later superceded by the Renal Physicians Association. This latter group, which came to have a leadership much broader than the original composition of the Friday-the-13th group, did incorporate as a private, not-for-profit organization. It did not seek Sec. 501(c) (3) tax-exempt status, however, in order to be free to represent its members' interests regarding the implementation of the ESRD program to both Congress and the executive branch.

A more direct protest against the interim regulations was the legal action initiated by nephrologists in New Jersey and California against the Secretary of HEW. A group of physicians in each of these states communicated extensively with various officials of HEW by means of personal visits, correspondence, and telephone calls, all extending over the period from July 1973 through February 1974. Members of the bureaucracy responded by internally debating the idea of a "retainer" or a capitation-fee basis for reimbursement. The two physician groups were assured in late November by the BHI that an intermediary letter establishing the option of a retainer concept was ready to be issued. In January, however, HEW first indicated it had rejected the retainer concept and then indicated it had made no decisions and was still considering

---

[n]Although little data is publicly available on the proprietary chains, a series of articles in the *Boston Globe* in 1971 discussed the development of the Babcock Artificial Kidney Center, the initial center of the National Medical Care/Biomedical Applications, Inc. chain, and its relation to the renal unit at Peter Bent Brigham Hospital, Boston. See the following by Richard A. Knox: "Brigham's Kidney Center Run for Profit," July 11; "Kidney Patients Plead for Life of Center," July 14; "M.D. in U.S. Plan Has Stake in Profit-making Kidney Units," July 25; "Brigham Permitted to Farm Out Work," September 15; "Kidney Pact Violated, Council Says," October 20. Other articles ran in the *Globe* on July 25, 26, and 30, 1971.

various options.[o] Exasperated after eight months of unsatisfactory petitioning of the government, the New Jersey group filed suit against the HEW Secretary in the U.S. District Court in Newark on March 4, 1974.[p]

Action inside HEW moved ahead, stimulated by the impending legal action. By early April, the decision had been made to permit physician reimbursement either through the provider facility, as initially specified, or directly to the physician on a retainer-concept basis. Physicians were required to be uniform in their preferences within a facility; that is, all physicians associated with a given provider facility could be reimbursed in one way only, although they had the choice of determining which way that was to be. Secretary of HEW Casper Weinberger announced this modification in the physician reimbursement procedure in New York City, April 17, 1974, in a final policies statement.[21]

The amount of capitation or retainer fee allowed by the intermediary letter of June 1974 that implemented the secretary's announced decision was a minimum of $160 and a maximum of $240 per patient per month.[22] Facility reimbursement screens were adjusted accordingly in those instances where physicians indicated a desire to be billed on the retainer basis.

Under the interim regulations, where payment of physician services was made by the provider facility, the effect was to establish a system of mandatory assignment of patient insurance benefits to the physician through the facility. That is, the facility, as a condition of participation, agreed to accept the established reimbursement rate for the dialysis procedure and to bill the program rather than the patient for services provided. The physician had no option but to acquiesce in the arrangement. When the alternative form of physician reimbursement was established by the final policies, this technically gave the physician the option of accepting or rejecting on a voluntary basis the assignment of patient benefits to him. Acceptance of voluntary assignment by the physician meant that he agreed to the established reimbursement rate and would bill the program rather than the patient. Rejection of assignment meant that the physician could bill the patient directly for services at any rate he desired. But the final policies clearly and forcefully indicated to the physician

[o]There are strong indications of fairly intense internal HEW discussion of the issues and their implications. The memorandum cited in reference note 17, page 236, stated: "While it is clear that the AMA has been opposed to any mechanism other than unit 'fee-for-service,' nephrologists have expressed both interest and support." A memorandum of March 8, 1974, added that "the AMA recently has limited their objection to any mechanism that established rigid fees": see Memorandum, From Director, Office of Health Financing Policy Development, To Assistant Secretary for Health, "Kidney Disease Treatment Program of Medicare—Reimbursement Policy Issues—INFORMATION," December 19, 1973, revised January 4, 1974, revised February 12, 1974, revised March 8, 1974, p. 13.

[p]See New York State Renal Physicians Association, Newsletter, March 7, 1974, pp. 5–8, for a summary of the activity of the New Jersey group. See also Sam J. Scaiella et al., Plaintiffs vs. Casper W. Weinberger et al., Defendants, United States District Court for the District of New Jersey, March 4, 1974.

community that failure to accept voluntary assignment of patient benefits could well result in the establishment of a mandatory assignment requirement.[23]

We do not have data that would indicate the impact of the alternative physician reimbursement method on the total costs of the program or on incentives to contain costs. But we may make several observations about the problems of regulating the costs of medical services through controls on physician reimbursement. First, a sweeping revision of fee-for-service reimbursement of physicians is probably impossible under even the most favorable of situations. Second, modifications of fee-for-service payment in the direction of retainer or capitation fees might lead to a split between the American Medical Association and medical specialty groups, depending on the particular medical specialty. Third, the presence of a substantial number of salaried physicians among the total physician population might ease the modification of physician reimbursement procedures in the direction of a cost-reducing arrangement. Finally, the design of incentives for economy and efficiency in the delivery of medical services, as a matter of simple prudence, must allow for the significant effect that both the contingency and the threat of litigation have on policy.

Unaddressed Cost-Control Issues

There are at least two issues of a clinical nature that strongly affect the ESRD program's costs but that have not been addressed in the interim program. The first is patient-selection criteria, and the second is the modality of treatment for the dialysis patient.

Patient-Selection Criteria. Hemodialysis was established as a therapy through a process of selecting the most medically suitable patients for treatment. Gradually, as experience developed in treating ESRD patients, first age criteria were relaxed and then criteria pertaining to other complicating medical problems were also relaxed. In the current context, in which financial barriers to treatment have been removed, we are witnessing what one physician calls "diminished contraindications for therapy." In other words, there are fewer and fewer clinical reasons to deny therapy to an individual able to benefit from it in even a small way. The consequence is that many centers are seeing the marginal patient become an increasing proportion of their total patient population. Overall estimates of the ESRD beneficiaries, therefore, tend to be biased downward because this dynamic is either overlooked or its implications are difficult to estimate. Total program costs, quite obviously, are pushed upward by this phenomenon. Moreover, the recent General Accounting Office report reflects the pressures generated by the public for establishing uniformity of patient selection criteria by liberalizing these criteria.[q]

Modality of Treatment. The most recent and best available data on dialysis costs indicates that cost is primarily sensitive to the location of treatment.[24] In-center (or hospital) dialysis is more expensive than limited-care dialysis, which, in turn, is more expensive than home dialysis. The critical variable, of course, is the medical and health professional's time. One of the more interesting aspects of the ESRD experience is that Medicare coverage of home dialysis, which is administered under Part B, does not cover all the expenses that are covered if an individual is dialyzed within an institution. The SSA has recognized this somewhat ironic situation, but has pointed out that changes in the law will be required before it can be responsive to the problem. Those changes have been proposed in legislation (S. 1492) introduced this past April by Senator Russell B. Long (D-La.). Similar legislation is also being considered by the House Ways and Means Committee.[25] In the meantime the ESRD program has been implemented in a way that provides no financial incentives for choosing home dialysis instead of institutional dialysis and actually provides disincentives to home dialysis. Such are the problems of incorporating a new program into the standard operating procedures of an established program.

Tentative Lessons from the ESRD Program Experience

It is far too early to draw definitive conclusions from the experience of the ESRD program. More extensive quantitative analysis of the actual experience of the program is obviously required. But there are a few tentative lessons that may be extracted:

1. Cost control is an instrumental objective of program implementation, which is *secondary* to the basic purpose of providing ESRD services.
2. The design phase of implementation is crucial for cost control since the subsequent problems of implementation emphasize routine processing of a highly administrative nature. Cost control is not the dominant administrative concern of implementation.
3. Bureaucratic competition and conflict between the SSA's BHI and the Office of the Assistant Secretary for Health of HEW will strongly affect cost-control design. BHI is likely to favor cost-control mechanisms that incorporate

---

[q]Comptroller General of the United States, *Treatment of Chronic Kidney Failure: Dialysis, Transplant, Costs, and the Need for More Vigorous Efforts* (Department of Health, Education, and Welfare), Washington, D.C., U.S. General Accounting Office, June 24, 1975, p. 54, recommended that the secretary should encourage "liberalized treatment criteria at facilities not accepting patients because of age, suitability for home dialysis, and diabetes and other diseases by establishing guidelines for treatment under Medicare."

administrative simplicity and maximum consistency with existing Medicare procedures. The Office of the Assistant Secretary is more likely to be concerned with an overall cost-control strategy, although it is also susceptible to the representation of other interests.

4. The design and execution of cost-control strategies for national health-insurance programs require some rationalization of the relations between the "insurance company" resources of BHI and the medical resources of the "health" side of HEW.

5. Cost-control and general program-design efforts involved in the financing of medical services will take place in a context in which the threat of litigation is ever present. The threat, moreover, will tend to induce conservative interpretations of close cases by administrators confronting the possibility of going to court over their decision. These contingencies cannot be avoided. They constitute an important aspect in the distribution of rights.

6. Regulation of medical services cannot move too far from the prevailing medical consensus in imposing cost-control constraints. It is not always easy to determine what the clinical consensus is, especially in something as complex as end-stage renal disease. The "best" clinical practice can be imposed as the norm only if a substantial minority supports that definition of "best."

7. The existence of a salaried physician population as a significant proportion of the total physican population can be regarded by the government as advantageous to cost control. Such physicians have no financial stake in defending fee-for-service; they may also be more sensitive to institutional needs for efficiency in the allocation of scarce resources.

8. Screens or ceilings on reimbursable expenses constitute a reasonably effective means for controlling costs. Such screens will be most effective where the medical procedures to which they are applied are relatively homogeneous in nature. Screens, as administered under ESRD Medicare, offer no incentive to a provider to charge at lesser rates.

9. There are likely to be a number of key variables affecting cost that are medical or clinical in nature, such as patient-selection criteria or modality of treatment. If these variables are defined primarily as clinical, public officials are likely to regard them as beyond the boundaries of legitimate government action.[r] Physicians are highly likely to regard government regulation of such variables as government interference in the practice of medicine. The policy

---

[r]It is precisely this position that was adopted recently by the Republican members of the Subcommittee on Oversight of the House Ways and Means Committee. "The Social Security Administration," they wrote, "should not set a 'norm', or even a goal for what is basically and most clearly a medical determination. Even though home dialysis is less costly than treatment in an institution, it should be left entirely up to the physicians and the patient to determine the best treatment alternative." See p. 18 of the *Report on Administration by the Social Security Administration of the End-Stage Renal Disease Program Established by Public Law 92-603 and On Social Security Medicare Research Studies,* cited in reference note 25, page 000.

toward such variables may have substantial cost implications.

10. The design of incentives to simultaneously promote the delivery of medical services and control the costs of those services remains a highly complex task.

4

Drug-Cost Control: The Road to Maximum Allowable-Cost Regulations

Thomas R. Fulda

After two years of debate involving the federal government, pharmaceutical manufacturers, and retail pharmacy groups, Secretary of Health, Education and Welfare Caspar Weinberger signed the Maximum Allowable Cost Regulations on July 25, 1975. Applicable to prescription drugs purchased directly by HEW or its contractors, and to drugs dispensed under departmental reimbursement programs, these regulations limit payments for designated multiple-source drugs to "the lowest unit price at which the drug is widely and consistently available from any formulator or labeler."[1] This limit is the maximum-allowable cost for the multiple-source drugs to which it is applied. The regulations also establish an upper limit to be set by the states, which is applicable to single as well as multiple-source drugs (including the MAC-listed drugs) dispensed in outpatient settings under HEW reimbursement programs. This upper limit is "the state's closest estimate of the price generally and currently paid by providers" plus a dispensing fee established by the state.[2] The significance of the MAC regulations is that they constitute the first attempt by the federal government to place specific limits on the amount that will be paid for drugs dispensed under HEW's reimbursement programs. When one is reminded that the issuance of these regulations occurred after more than 15 years of congressional investigations of the pharmaceutical industry *and* some ten years after the initial large-scale involvement of the federal government in the financing of health-care delivery through the Medicare and Medicaid programs, some of the complexities involved in attempting to control drug costs begin to appear.

Investigating the Pharmaceutical Industry

Since 1959 the United States Senate has undertaken three major investigations of the pharmaceutical industry and the Department of Health, Education and Welfare, a fourth one. Beginning in late 1959 Senator Estes Kefauver chaired the first of nearly three years of hearings on the drug industry held before the Senate Subcommittee on Antitrust and Monopoly.[3] Following the death of Senator Kefauver, and pointing to the need to "provide some better answers to important issues still in controversy," Senator Gaylord Nelson in May 1967 opened new hearings on the drug industry before the Subcommittee on Monopoly of the Senate Select Committee on Small Business.[4] Reacting to the passage two years earlier of a Medicare program that did not provide outpatient prescription-drug coverage, President Johnson ordered a comprehensive study of the cost of providing drug coverage under Medicare. The HEW Task Force on Prescription Drugs, which resulted from President Johnson's order, also began operations in May 1967.[5] Although the task force completed its work in 1969, both the Nelson hearings and hearings begun in 1973 before the Senate Health Subcommittee chaired by Senator Edward Kennedy are still continuing.

Prices and Profits

A full review of the findings of these investigations is beyond the scope of this study. A brief look, however, at what has been learned about drug prices is necessary for an understanding of the MAC regulations. As the congressional hearings progressed it quickly became clear that a central characteristic of the pharmaceutical marketplace is the absence of price competition in a large part of it. The lack of price competition in the pharmaceutical market is largely attributable to the patent system operating in this country. Under this system the holder of a patent is given exclusive rights over his discovery for 17 years.[6] As a result, the majority of the most frequently prescribed drugs are available from only one manufacturer.[a] Uninfluenced by the existence of other manufacturers of the same chemical entity, prices of single-source drugs are usually set at a level that bears little relationship to the manufacturer's production cost. With the help of liberal expenditures for advertising and promotion directed at the physician, because he decides what drug the consumer receives, those prices are often maintained at that level for periods well beyond the expiration of the drug's patent.[7]

Although patent monopolies and forms of nonprice competition dominate a large part of the pharmaceutical market, there is a small but growing segment of it where price competition does occur. In this so-called generic market, because patents have expired, cross-licensing has occurred, or for other reasons, the same chemical entity is available from a number of different firms at widely different prices. This market was once the province of small manufacturers but growing interest in generic prescribing has encouraged major manufacturers to enter it in recent years. Some examples of these price differences taken from the *Drug Topics Red Book*, a publication widely used by retail pharmacies, are shown in table 4-1. Manufacturers of the major brands of these multiple-source drugs have tried to justify their prices by arguing that their concern for quality results in a better product and by arguing that two chemically identical drugs may not be therapeutically equivalent and should not be used interchangeably unless equivalence can be established. The finding of the HEW

---

[a]In 1974 approximately 25 percent of the most frequently prescribed drugs to outpatients were available from more than one manufacturer.

Table 4-1
Multiple-Source Drug-Price Comparisons

Product	Price Major Brand	Price Generic
Propoxyphene HCL 65 mg 100	$7.02 Darvon Eli Lilly	$3.60 SK-65 Smith Klein Corp.
Meprobamate 400 mg 100's	$6.00 Equanil Wyeth	$1.49 Kessobamate McKesson Pharmaceuticals
Reserpine .25 mg 1000	$39.50 Serpasil Ciba	$9.76 Sandril Eli Lilly
Nitrofurantoin 50 mg 100	$10.26 Furandantin Eaton Laboratories	$1.75 Nitrofurantoin Ketchum Labs.
Sulfisoxazole .5 gm 1000	$26.60 Gantrisin Roche	$10.64 Sulfisoxazole Purepac

Source: *Drug Topics Red Book* (Oradell, N.J.: Medical Economics Company, 1976).

Task Force on Prescription Drugs and testimony by the commissioner of the Food and Drug Administration before the Senate Small Business Committee have not supported these assertions.[8]

Criticism of drug price levels, and of price variations within and between segments of the pharmaceutical market, which result from the absence of price competition, has frequently been coupled with attacks on the high level of pharmaceutical industry profits. The drug industry has a long record of high profitability. Annual *Fortune* magazine rankings of major industrial corporations by net after-tax profit on invested capital has frequently found drug firms high on the list. Comparison (table 4-2) on the average net profit after taxes (as a

Table 4-2
Average Net Profits after Taxes as a Percentage of Net Stockholders' Equity, U.S. Drug Manufacturers and All U.S. Manufacturing Corporations

Year	Drug Manufacturers	All Manufacturers
1960	17.0%	9.3%
1965	20.5	13.1
1970	18.2	9.4
1971	19.3	9.7
1972	18.8	10.7
1973	19.0	12.9
1974	18.8	15.1

Source: *Quarterly Financial Report for Manufacturing Corporations,* FTC-SEC.

percent of stockholders equity) of United States drug manufacturers with the rate for all United States manufacturing corporations shows that profits for drug firms have been consistently above those for all manufacturing corporations.

To justify its prices and its profits, representatives of the pharmaceutical industry have frequently argued that high earnings levels are necessary to support high levels of research and development expenditures without which the flow of new drug discoveries would cease. Although it is true that the pharmaceutical industry spends considerable sums on research and has produced important therapeutic advances, there is some evidence suggesting that the importance of the results of pharmaceutical industry research has been overstated. The HEW task force found that "important new chemical entities represent only a fraction—perhaps 10 to 25 percent of all new products introduced each year and the remainder consists merely of minor modifications or combination products," and concluded as a result that "much of the drug industry's research and development activities would appear to provide only minor contributions to medical progress."[9]

Minimal Results

Although Congress has devoted much effort to investigations of the drug industry, attempts to pass legislation that would reduce drug prices have been unsuccessful. The Kefauver hearings did result in the passage of the Kefauver-Harris Amendments in 1962. They require that a new drug must be proven efficacious for the conditions for which it is recommended before the Food and Drug Administration will clear it for marketing.[10] Opposed by the AMA and the Pharmaceutical Manufacturers Association as well as a powerful group of adversaries in the Senate, which included Senators Dirkson, Hruska and Eastland, final passage of the Kefauver-Harris Amendments was due at least in part to the story of the thalidomide tragedy, which became known during consideration of the legislation.[11] Provisions of the amendments that would have required compulsory patent licensing of drug products were striken prior to final passage of the legislation. In recent years Senator Nelson has introduced legislation to ban the use of brand names, to require compulsory patent licensing, and to reform other industry practices, but to date final action by Congress has not been taken on any of these bills.[b]

---

[b]94th Congress 1st Session: S 1312 would require mandatory patent licensing under certain conditions and S 1324 would prohibit the use of any name in connection with any prescription drug other than the official name for such drug. See also S 1313, 1314, 1315, 1316, 1317, 1318, 1319, 1320, 1321, 1322, 1323, 1325, and 2621.

Cost-Control Pressures—A New Focus

Although Congress has not dealt with the drug-price issue, consideration of the health-care cost problem, of which drugs are a small part, has taken on new importance as a result of increased federal involvement in the financing of health-care delivery. This involvement began with passage of Title XVIII (Medicare) and XIX (Medicaid) of the Social Security Act in 1965. Government spending for these programs helped to fuel rapid increases in health-care costs, which have outstripped the general level of inflation the country has experienced. The rate of increase in medical-care prices is compared with the rate of increase for all goods and services in table 4-3. Increasing health-care expenditures have in turn been reflected in higher costs for health-care programs financed by the government. Table 4-4 compares total national health-care expenditures with expenditures for health services and supplies under Medicare and Medicaid. Between fiscal years 1967 and 1974, expenditures for Medicare and Medicaid have increased from $5.9 to $22.5 billion. Concern over rising program costs led to the passage in late 1972 of HR 1, which became Public Law 92-603. This law places upper limits on reasonable physician charges, puts an upper limit on reasonable hospital charges, and establishes Professional Standards Review Organizations to review the quality and necessity of services provided under government programs.

Just as rising health-care costs and rising program expenditures precipitated growing interest in cost control, rising expenditures for prescription drugs (about 10 percent of total health expenditures) and rising costs of

Table 4-3
Health-Care Price Increases

Year	Average Annual Percentage Increase	
	CPI (All Items)	(Medical Care)
1950–55	2.2	3.8
1955–60	2.0	4.1
1960–65	1.3	2.5
1965–70	4.2	6.1
1971	4.3	6.5
1972	3.3	3.2
1973	6.2	3.9
1974	11.0	9.3

Source: *Medical Care Expenditures, Prices and Costs: Background Book* Social Security Administration, September 1975.

Table 4-4
Health-Care Expenditures: Medicare and Medicaid
(in Millions)

Fiscal Year	National Health Expenditures	Medicare Expenditures	Medicaid[a] Expenditures
1967	$ 47,879	$ 3,395	$ 2,475
1968	53,765	5,347	3,723
1969	60,617	6,598	4,596
1970	69,202	7,149	5,213
1971	77,162	7,875	6,278
1972	86,687	8,819	7,752
1973	95,384	9,479	9,209
1974	104,030	11,322	11,218

Source: Compendium of national health expenditures data, Social Security Administration, January 1976; and "National Health Expenditures, Fiscal Year 1975," Marjorie Smith Mueller and Robert M. Gibson, *Social Security Bulletin*, February 1976.

[a]Includes both federal and state expenditures under Title XIX.

providing drug coverage under Medicare[c] and Medicaid[d] precipitated new interest in controlling drug costs. Table 4-5 charts the growth in expenditures for drugs and drug sundries as well as the growth in expenditures for these items under Medicare and Medicaid beginning with fiscal year 1967.[e]

---

[c]Medicare, administered by the Social Security Administration, is a two-part program designed to make sure that senior citizens who are faced with greater health needs and declining or fixed incomes receive adequate health care. Part A of the program, which is financed by deductions from employee wages and taxes on employers, provides hospitalization insurance, which includes prescription-drug coverage for drugs dispensed in hospitals and nursing homes. Part B of the program, which is financed by monthly premiums paid by program beneficiaries, provides supplementary medical insurance for physicians services, x-rays, and so on, but *not* for out-of-hospital prescription drugs.

[d]Medicaid, administered by each state under the supervision of HEW's Social and Rehabilitation Service, provides medical assistance to the blind, the aged, the disabled, and families with dependent children. The standard benefit package provided by each state includes inpatient and outpatient hospital care, physicians' services, nursing-home care, and so on. Prescription-drug coverage is provided to the recipients of benefits while inpatients in hospitals or nursing homes, and, *unlike Medicare,* outpatient drugs are provided at the option of each state. Only three states (Alaska, Oklahoma, and Wyoming) do not provide some form of out-of-hospital prescription drug benefit. Funding for Medicaid programs is provided by the states with the federal government participating on a cost-sharing basis.

[e]The category *drugs and drug sundries* includes prescription-drugs pharmaceutical products not requiring a prescription and other over-the-counter health items. No figures are available that isolate prescription-drug expenditures from other products included in this category.

Table 4-5
Expenditures for Drugs and Drug Sundries
(in Millions)

| Fiscal Year | National Expenditures | Total Medicare and Medicaid | Medicare Institutional[a] | Medicaid[b] | |
				Institutional[a]	Outpatient
1967	$5,480	$ 599.0	$ 247.9	$159.5	$191.5
1968	5,865	842.4	364.5	227.4	250.5
1969	6,482	1,042.1	461.5	265.0	315.6
1970	7,114	1,207.8	498.8	298.8	410.2
1971	7,626	1,439.9	560.9	393.3	505.2
1972	8,233	1,704.4	633.3	505.2	565.9
1973	8,987	1,914.9	688.9	563.5	662.5
1974	9,612	2,150.5	819.1	625.0	706.4

Source: Thomas R. Fulda, *Prescription Drug Data Summary,* 1974, Department of Health, Education and Welfare, Publication SSA 76-11928.

[a]Estimates institutional drug expenditures at 10 percent of hospital expenditures and 7 percent of nursing-home costs.

[b]Includes both federal and state funds.

Approaches to Drug-Cost Control

To cope with rising drug expenditures and the increasing cost of providing prescription-drug coverage under Medicare and Medicaid, attention has been focused primarily on two approaches to controlling drug costs. One approach involves the use of utilization review techniques to assess the quality of drug therapy that is provided and to determine the impact on drug costs of improvements in such therapy. The other approach involves efforts to make reimbursement mechanisms under present and contemplated programs for providing prescription drug benefits more cost effective.

Quality of Care and Program Cost

Assessing the link between drug therapy and its cost involves answering three questions. Are patients getting the right drug for the right condition in the right amounts at the right time? If not, what should be done to improve the quality of care? How will improvements in the quality of care influence the cost of providing care? Utilization review using electronic data-processing techniques provides a means for answering these questions. Through utilization review it is possible to determine what drugs are being prescribed by individual physicians, dispensed by particular pharmacies, and used by individual patients.

Studies of drug use have indicated there is some cause for concern about the quality of drug therapy. A study by the San Joaquin Medical Foundation Drug Program involving 50,000 people showed that 7.6 percent of those receiving prescriptions were receiving drugs that interact with other drugs they were using.[12] Another study conducted by Dr. Louis Lasagna and some colleagues compared the use of three drugs (cephalexin, allopurinol, and propranolol HCL) for hospitalized patients with the labeling recommendation for them approved by the Food and Drug Administration.[13] Each of the drugs was prescribed frequently for therapeutic indications not mentioned in the approved labeling. The authors found that since the FDA-approved labeling agreed with current medical literature, prescribing of the drugs for other conditions was inappropriate.

Although experts may disagree about its extent there is little doubt that irrational prescribing is occurring and that it has significant economic consequences.[f] Writing in the *New England Journal of Medicine,* Dr. Kenneth Melmon has suggested that increased use of medical-care resources is one consequence of improper prescribing. Dr. Melmon indicated that 18 to 30 percent of all hospitalized patients have a drug reaction, and that the duration of their hospitalization is about doubled as a consequence. In addition, 3 to 5 percent of all admissions to hospitals are primarily for drug reactions.[14] As a result, Dr. Melmon suggests, about one-seventh of all hospital days are devoted to the care of drug toxicity. Dr. Robert Maronde in a study *Drug Utilization Review With On Line Computer Capability* published in 1972 concluded that improvements in the quality of drug therapy through effective utilization review programs would reduce prescription-drug costs a minimum of 14 percent.[15]

Cost-Effective Reimbursement Mechanisms

Efforts to improve the cost-effectiveness of reimbursement mechanisms used to provide prescription-drug benefits have concentrated on attempts to determine the most cost-effective approach to the provision of prescription-drug benefits under future programs (outpatient drug benefits under Medicare or drug benefits under national health insurance); to develop alternative reimbursement approaches that could be used under existing programs; and to improve the cost-effectiveness of existing reimbursement mechanisms under present programs providing prescription drug coverage.

To determine the most cost-effective approach to providing prescription-drug benefits under future programs the Department of Health, Education and Welfare began funding in 1975 a contract to measure the effect of various

---

[f]For a different view of the problem see Lee, Armistead M., *Drug Use Data: A Different Perspective*, JAMA Vol. 234, No. 12, December 22, 1975, pp. 124–44.

proposed drug-benefit cost-sharing alternatives on both program and administrative costs. Although Medicare does not now cover outpatient prescription drugs, four outpatient-benefit packages were developed for a sample of Medicare beneficiaries in California and the beneficiaries have been assigned randomly to one of the benefit programs. Some beneficiaries receive free drugs, others pay $1 per prescription, and still others pay 25 percent of the price of each prescription. A fourth group must meet a $50 deductible and then pay 25 percent of the cost of each prescription after the deductible has been met. Results of this experiment will be available beginning late in 1976.

As an alternative to the existing reimbursement methods used under its Medicaid program the State of California is considering a volume purchase plan.[16] If this plan is adopted, instead of paying the provider of services (the pharmacist) his cost to purchase the drug plus a charge for dispensing it, the state will let competitive bids and obtain drugs at the best price it can get consistent with the purchasing power that results from quantity buying. Under this plan, which would at first be limited to 75 multiple-source drugs, the state would pay wholesalers to distribute the drugs to retail pharmacies and, as before, would pay retail pharmacists a fee to fill Medicaid prescriptions.

The Maximum Allowable-Cost Regulations

Interest in improving the cost-effectiveness of existing reimbursement mechanisms for providing drug benefits under the Medicare and Medicaid programs led Secretary Caspar Weinberger to announce on December 19, 1973 before the Senate Health Subcommittee that HEW would propose regulations "to limit drug reimbursements under programs administered by the Department to the lowest cost at which the drug is generally available unless there is a demonstrated difference in therapeutic effect."[17] During the 11 intervening months between this announcement and the publication of the proposed Maximum Allowable Cost Regulations in the *Federal Register* on November 15, 1974, two things happened.[18] Within HEW efforts were made with the consultation of pharmacy, drug industry, physicians groups, and others to translate the Secretary's policy pronouncement into publishable regulations. Outside the department an old question resurfaced: To what extent can chemically equivalent drug products produced by different manufacturers be substituted for each other without a change in the therapeutic effect that is produced.

Opponents of the MAC regulations argued that unless two chemically identical drugs prove to be bioequivalent they cannot be presumed to produce the same therapeutic effect and should not be used interchangeably as might result from the implementation of the regulations. Two drugs are bioequivalent if the extent to which and the rate at which their active ingredients are absorbed into the blood are similar. Proponents of the MAC regulations argued that bioequivalent drugs are not necessarily therapeutically inequivalent. They defended FDA quality and bioequivalence standards as adequate to ensure the quality of drugs on the market and to deal with the bioequivalence problem to the extent that it exists.[19]

Faced with these divergent viewpoints expressed during hearings before the Senate Health Subcommittee, Senator Kennedy referred the matter to the newly created Office of Technology Assessment for review. In July 1974 a study panel headed by Dr. Robert Berliner, M.D., Dean of the Yale University School of Medicine, issued its *Drug Bioequivalence* report.[20] Describing the findings of the report during testimony before the Subcommittee on Monopoly of the Senate Small Business Committee, Dr. Berliner indicated that the panel "concluded that there are at least some categories of drug products for which it will be necessary to establish adequate bioavailability standards before interchangeability could even be considered." He continued that "drugs for which direct demonstration of bioavailability would be necessary constitute a small minority of all drugs" and concluded that it would be possible to develop a list of drugs that could be considered interchangeable because proof of bioequivalence would not be considered necessary.[21] Although the Pharmaceutical Manufacturers Association concluded that the Office of Technology Assessment report vindicated its anti-MAC position, HEW concluded that nothing in the report justified a delay in issuing the MAC regulations.[22]

After reviewing more than 2,000 comments on the proposed regulations, most of which contained negative reaction from individuals and groups affected by them, the final Maximum Allowable Cost Regulations were published by HEW in the *Federal Register* of July 31, 1975.[23] They contain two major provisions.

First, reimbursements for multiple-source drugs "for which significant amounts of Federal funds are or may be expended" will be limited "to the lowest unit price at which the drug is widely and consistently available from any formulator or labeler."[24] This limit is the maximum-allowable cost for the multiple-source drugs to which it is applied. Setting an upper limit on what will be paid for multiple-source drugs is a recognition by HEW of increased generic prescribing and an attempt by the department to take advantage of price competition existing in the multiple-source drug market. As table 4-6 indicates, generic prescribing has been steadily increasing for the last ten years. Multiple-source drugs, which, as table 4-1 indicates, are frequently available at widely different prices, account for approximately 25 percent of the 200 most frequently prescribed drugs in the outpatient market. As patents expire in the next several years a number of large-selling single-source drugs will become part of the multiple-source drug market.

To select drugs to which MAC limits will be applicable the regulations establish a Pharmaceutical Reimbursement Board and a Pharmaceutical Reimbursement Advisory Committee. The board is composed of 6 full-time HEW

Table 4-6
New Generic Prescriptions as a
Percentage of Total New Rx's

Year	Percentage
1966	6.4
1967	7.0
1968	8.2
1969	8.8
1970	9.0
1971	9.2
1972	9.7
1973	10.6
1974	10.7
1975	11.1

Source: *Pharmacy Times*, April 1976.

employees and the advisory committee of 15 nongovernment experts in pharmacy, pharmacology, medicine, pharmaceutical marketing, public health, and consumer affairs.

The process of selecting multiple-source drugs, which will have MAC limits set on them, begins with the identification by the Pharmaceutical Reimbursement Board of multiple-source drugs that will provide savings to HEW if reimbursement limits are set on them. The selection criteria used are the spread in prices among producers of a given drug and the size of HEW expenditures for it. For drugs identified as offering significant savings potential, the Food and Drug Administration will be asked by the board to determine if there are any pending regulatory actions, quality or bioequivalency problems, that would make it unwise to establish a MAC limit. If FDA does not determine that no MAC limit should be set, this means FDA believes that all suppliers of the drug in question engaged in interstate commerce meet official standards necessary to market the drug; meet bioequivalency standards if applicable; have had a recent plant inspection by FDA; and meet other tests imposed by the FDA. A *proposed* MAC limit is then set on that drug and published in the *Federal Register*.

After publication of the proposed MAC limit the board submits its decisions to the Pharmaceutical Reimbursement Advisory Committee for review. The committee, whose findings are published, may delay, modify, or approve the actions of the board. After considering the committee's recommendations the board then publishes a MAC limit in the *Federal Register*. Unless new evidence is presented during a 30-day comment period or as a result of administrative hearings, which may be requested, the MAC limit becomes final and remains in effect until reconsidered by the board.

There is one exception to the applicability of a MAC limit to a specific multiple-source drug. If a physician states in his own handwriting that a particular brand of given chemical entity is medically necessary, then reimbursement under HEW programs will be paid for a brand of the drug that is higher in price than the MAC limit.

The second part of the MAC regulations involves changes in the way reimbursements are made under outpatient Medicaid drug programs. Until this change most states and many nongovernment third-party programs reimbursed out-of-hospital providers on the basis of published average wholesale prices. Since, according to data provided by the pharmaceutical industry, these published prices overstate actual prices paid by the pharmacist by an average of 15 to 18 percent, future outpatient Medicaid reimbursements for single and multiple-source drugs will now be limited to the lower of the estimated acquisition cost plus a dispensing fee or the provider's usual and customary charge to the general public.[25]

To assist the states in arriving at their best estimate of the actual cost to the pharmacist of outpatient drugs dispensed under Medicaid, as is required by the MAC regulations, HEW has agreed to provide price information on the cost of frequently prescribed drugs. In addition, since under the regulations the pharmacist must be paid a fee related to the cost of filling a prescription, the states will be required to conduct surveys of pharmacy operating costs.

Reimbursing pharmacists on the basis of estimated acquisition cost plus a dispensing fee has resulted in a considerable degree of dissatisfaction with the MAC regulations among retail pharmacists. The prospect of being deprived of the difference between the actual cost of a drug to the retailer and the higher average wholesale cost, which now provides the basis for his Medicaid reimbursement for the drug, has brought forth increased demands for adjustment upward of the dispensing fee. Although the MAC regulations require that the pharmacist be paid a fee based on periodic surveys of pharmacy operating costs for filling Medicaid prescriptions, fee setting is legally the responsibility of each state, and there is some question whether or not the pharmacist will receive the fee adjustment they are seeking. Since Medicaid dispensing fees are set subject to the budgetary constraints that each state must face, should fee surveys determine that increases are in order, whether or not they will be granted may depend as much on budget limitations as on questions of equity.

To supplement these efforts to make HEW drug-reimbursement programs more cost-effective, efforts are also underway to develop a prescription drug-price publication for distribution to physicians and consumers. This publication will list the most frequently prescribed drugs and display prices generally paid by the pharmacist for them in such a way as to facilitate easy comparison of the different prices at which a given drug is available from its producers. It is hoped that making prescription-price information available to physicians, who decide what drugs the consumer purchases, will encourage greater cost consciousness in prescribing and dispensing decisions and will result in a reduction in the cost of drugs for the consumer without any sacrifice in the quality of patient care.

The Next Phase

The road toward establishing the Maximum Allowable Cost regulations has been long and sometimes tortuous. Although the regulations have been issued, it is difficult to predict the extent to which they will accomplish their intended objective. Legal challenges to the regulations filed by the American Medical Association and others are still to be resolved.[26] Whether or not the regulations will actually result in a net $55 to 70 million savings in the cost of providing prescription drugs under Medicare and Medicaid, as originally estimated by HEW, will have to be shown.[g]

Although questions surround the future of the Maximum Allowable Cost regulations, a change in thinking about health-care cost controls and drug-cost control in particular is clearly discernible. In the mid-1960's Medicare and Medicaid may have been enacted without the inclusion of adequate cost-control procedures, but the experience of the last ten years has linked together solving the cost problem and possibilities for the enactment of new health-care programs in the future. Commenting on the possibility that Medicare coverage might be expanded to provide outpatient prescription-drug benefits Senator Herman Talmadge, who chairs the Subcommittee on Health of the Senate Finance Committee said, "Until we can apply reasonable controls effectively in present programs, I don't see Congress adding benefits which can only add to our problem."[27] Commenting on the importance of the MAC regulations as a means of dealing with the drug cost-control problem *before* providing drug benefits under national health insurance becomes an issue, Secretary of Health, Education and Welfare Casper Weinberger made essentially the same point when he suggested that without limits on drug reimbursements, and incentives to use lower priced drugs, providing prescription drugs under national health insurance would be prohibitively expensive.

---

[g]For savings see Inflation Impact Statement on CFR 45, Subtitle A, Part 19, Limitations on Payments on Reimbursement for Drugs.

Part III

Health-Care Regulation: Defining Alternatives

5

Medical Politics and Medical Prices: The Relation between Who Decides and How Much it Costs

Jane Cassels Record

Speaking informally to a small group of health administrators in early 1976, a high-ranking economist in the federal bureaucracy said, "The plain fact is that medical costs are flat out of control—and there is no agreement on what to do about the situation."

The statement came as no surprise. With health goods and services exceeding 8 percent of the Gross National Product, with the federal government paying more than 40 percent of the nation's medical bill, and with the health industry helping to pace a startling upthrust in the Consumer Price Index, how to control prices and costs in the health-care sector had become one of the liveliest issues in American public policy.

Why had the price and cost situation gotten out of hand? The answer to that question, like the solution to the problem, is obviously complex. This chapter will explore one aspect of the problem: the relation between explosive medical prices and persistent ambiguities about how decisions concerning health issues should be made. The focus of the discourse can be summed in the following questions. Which matters should be decided by the government bureaucracy? Which should be assigned to market forces? Which should be left to the medical profession? What implications does the locus of decision have for medical prices? Issues to be decided include interrelated matters such as the price and quality of health goods and services, consumer access to knowledge, consumer access to care, the number and distribution of physicians, and consumer choice with respect to prepaid versus fee-for-service arrangements.

The three legislative areas singled out here—the Professional Standards Review Organization (PSRO), medical education, and the Health Maintenance Organization (HMO) Act—are not the only federal initiatives for dealing with the inadequacies of the traditional decision-making arrangements. The last 10 to 12 years have witnessed a freshet of Congressional activity in the health field, and implicit in virtually every instance has been the provocative question of who should decide what the price, content, availability, and delivery mechanism of health care should be. The PSRO, medical-education, and HMO initiatives illustrate particularly well the relation of decision locus or power distribution to rising prices and to cost containment.

Grateful acknowledgement is made to the many staff members of congressional committees and HEW agencies who have shared with the author their experiences, opinions, and documentary materials; special thanks go to Scott Fleming, Robert Knouss, Merwyn R. Greenlick, and Ernest W. Saward for valuable suggestions.

Although there are health professionals other than physicians, *profession* as used here refers to physicians unless otherwise stated, because the focus is upon medical prices and costs, and because the medical profession has dominated the health field. The term *medical*, when referring to price, cost, quality, and so on, describes primarily the kinds of services provided by physicians; the broader term *health* describes all the goods and services included in the national income accounts and in the Consumer Price Index as belonging roughly to the health industry.

Although the terms price and cost are often used interchangeably in literature about medical care, they are used more distinctively in this chapter. *Price* refers to the dollar amount for which an individual good or service is purchased. *Cost* is used to describe dollar payments to the factors of production in turning out the good or service. Thus the difference between average price and average cost is the firm's *rate of profit* (or *loss*). *Expenditures* is used here to describe the total amounts paid by the government or a health-insurance agency or a consumer for a bundle of goods and services. Expenditures thus are determined both by the prices of the individual goods and services in the bundle and by the size of the bundle. The "rising national medical expenditures," which have been paid with tax dollars, for example, are attributable not only to rising prices but also to larger volumes of goods and services purchased by the federal government during the past decade, particularly for the poor and elderly.

The Traditional Power Arrangements

A striking feature of national policy in the health field down through the decades has been government restraint. In spite of the critical importance of health care for the welfare of citizens individually and collectively, and in spite of the growing portion of the nation's health bill paid from tax revenues, there has been a persistent reluctance to socialize the health industry in whole or in part. As a general rule the provision of health services has been left to private initiative, organization, and ownership except for matters such as sanitation, where a critical service is virtually impossible to individualize and therefore must be purchased collectively. The very term "public health" has been associated primarily with just such kinds of services, as opposed to the diagnosis and treatment of disease, where services usually can be individualized and marketed for a profit.

The premise that the provision of personal medical care should be lodged in the private sector, except for a few special groups such as the armed forces and war veterans, has rested on the assumption that the market mechanism would serve the public interest in two primary ways: First, both within the medical industry and between it and other industries, market forces would allocate economic resources to produce a total bundle of goods and services that accorded more nearly with consumer preferences than would be the case if decisions about what to produce, how to produce it, at what price, and so on were made by government bureaucracy. Second, the market not only would privatize but also would decentralize decision-making power and ipso facto serve as a constraint upon the concentration of power in an ever-encroaching state. Unfortunately, there have been strong noncompetitive elements both in the market where factors of production (including physicians) are sold and in the market where goods and services are sold. Noncompetitive forces have been particularly strong on the supply side, and monopolistic elements tend to restrict output or *quantity* and to raise prices and costs. Look, for example, at the supply of physicians. The higher salaries, which employers of MDs had to pay, and the higher incomes, which self-employed MDs could earn, because members of the profession were scarce, should have induced more persons to enter the profession, with a dampening effect on salaries and incomes; but entry was controlled by the medical profession. In the product market, methods of organizing medical-care delivery, which appeared to be more efficient than the traditional fee-for-service practices, were opposed, with considerable success, by organized medicine through its primary voice, the American Medical Association (AMA). Even in a competitive market, *access* to care would be rationed by the price of medical goods and services. For those who could not pay the price, care would depend upon public or private charity, including the physician's willingness to reduce prices or omit bills for such patients.[a] The great shift from private to public subsidy as the dominant mode of providing medical services for the medically underserved was a hallmark of the 1960s.

What about *quality* of care? Traditionally quality assurance was an area of decision making ceded almost entirely to the medical profession. In discharging the quality-assurance obligation, as it was interpreted by the profession, organized medicine has directed its energies in large measure at controlling entry to the profession through medical-school requirements, qualifying examinations, and licensure procedures. Whether control of entry was prompted primarily by a concern for quality of care or by a concern for the economic interests of physicians is a controversial matter.[1] No doubt both motives were present. Those who would espouse quality assurance as the only dominant motive of the profession are confronted by the fact that not until the last few years have refresher courses or continuing education been required for license renewal;[b] moreover, the profession has exhibited strong reluctance to assume collective responsibility for the professional performance of individual

---

[a]For a discussion of physician charity as physician-serving price discrimination, see R.A. Kessel, "Price Discrimination in Medicine," *Journal of Law and Economics*, I (October, 1958), 20 ff.

[b]For a review of the licensure situation and an indication of congressional inclination, see Report 94-887, U.S. Senate Committee on Labor and Public Welfare, May, 1976, pp. 69–84.

physicians. Such reluctance is characteristic of professions in general.[2]

Extreme marketeers such as Milton Friedman have advocated the abolition of entry requirements. Physicians or others offering themselves as medical practitioners would be free to advertise their qualifications and prices, and consumers would be free to choose a health-care provider.[3] Organized medicine has opposed that kind of open competition in general and advertising in particular; indeed, prohibition of advertising has been written into state laws, at physician initiative, as unprofessional conduct even for the duly licensed practitioner. The Friedman approach essentially would assign quality assurance to the competitive market, along with decisions about price and quantity of service, the assumption being that provider competition and consumer knowledge would weed out incompetents.

Market, Profession, and the Public Interest

The state has the power to preempt decision making in virtually any or all matters relating to medical care. But in most areas, it has ceded authority to the market or the profession. This delegation of price and quality assurance does not rest on any *right*, nor on any intrinsic value of the market mechanism per se. The grant of authority to market and profession is defendable only on the postulate that such delegation serves the common good. Moreover, only if market and professional behaviors validate the postulate in an ongoing way is continued delegation justified. Thus to meet the test over time, market and profession must produce a better combination of prices, quantity of output, quality of service, and degree of choice or freedom than would be produced by other decision-making arrangements. What brings *market* behavior presumably into accord with the public interest is vigorous competition in both supply and demand. The supposed moderator of *professional* behavior, bringing it into consonance with the public interest, is the professional ethic. Because the stated public-interest regulator in each case—market or profession—is essentially internal, it until recently, at least, was widely assumed and proclaimed that no external regulation—for instance, from government—was necessary to protect consumer and citizen interests; indeed, from that point of view, interference from the outside was inherently, almost by definition, inimical to the common good.

The problem is that the internal regulators have not worked. Strong, persistent elements of monopoly have distorted market decisions about price and quantity, and in the quality area, organized medicine's[c] behavior often has been

---

[c]"Organized medicine," which refers to the American Medical Association or similar goal-oriented professional groupings, is different from the more general term "profession". One can be a member of the latter without affiliation with organized medicine.

physician or profession serving rather than consumer or public serving. Yet market or professional behavior, which has been questioned as antisocial or antipublic, or anticonsumer, is often defended by reference to market or profession as though they were talismen or first principles. But market and professional decisions are means rather than ends; the end is the public interest. Furthermore, when large amounts of public funds are entailed, decisions delegated to the private sector must be publicly accountable.

The physician who believes it is in the public interest for him to pursue his self-interest as a practicing entrepreneur or businessman inhabits the same skin as the physician who believes his motives must be above self-aggrandisement. The ambiguity of the two ethics is illustrated by the fact that it is the profession which, however motivated, has most effectively constrained competition in the market. Moreover, physician domination of decision making has extended far beyond the area of physician expertise,[4] intruding into questions of whether medical care should be prepaid, whether new hospitals should be built and in what location, and so on.

The Impact of Medicare and Medicaid

The dramatic, new federal initiatives of the middle 1960s, particularly Medicare and Medicaid, revealed the frailties of the allocation of power and the inadequacies of market and profession to effectuate national priorities as those priorities were being redefined. As part of this redefinition the Medicare and Medicaid acts were addressed to a quickening social perception of medical care as a right, to be underwritten by the public purse where necessary.

Responding to the plight of the indigent, Congress elected to purchase medical care in the private sector rather than through publicly owned delivery systems. In choosing that route and in failing to deal effectively and unambiguously in advance with conspicuous flaws in existing institutional arrangements, national policy makers courted disaster. In spite of a widely deplored, long-standing shortage of physicians and in spite of a virtual certainty that the elevation of demand brought on by Medicare and Medicaid would precipitate an up-push in prices, enriching physicians and other suppliers of goods and services in the health field at the expense of the taxpayers, Congress, under severe pressure from the AMA, declined to control physician fees—even temporarily—until the supply of physicians could be increased as a countervailing force in price determination. Moreover, the new acts placed control of utilization in the hands of the profession, in spite of the profession's demonstrated reluctance to discipline its members, however few, who violated the Hippocratic obligation to treat only where treatment is likely to improve the patient's health.

The result was skyrocketing prices, alleged frequent overutilization, costs which increasingly overran predictions, and widespread public indignation.

National policy makers, at least theoretically, had three alternative responses: to leave the existing instruments of decision basically intact; to socialize the medical-care industry; or to develop new forms of social control or regulation that would attempt to bring the performance of market and profession more closely into accord with stated public interests and priorities. The first alternative was politically untenable; the second, ideologically unacceptable. That left the third route, and much of the major legislation of recent years has purported to graft new positive or negative incentive arrangements, or new procedures and controls, onto the traditional market and professional institutions without destroying their force as primary shapers of medical-care content and organization in the United States.

This third route still offered a wide range of options in dealing with market and profession. With respect to the market, two distinctive strategies were available: (1) accept the market as noncompetitive and regulate its decisions or (2) regulate or manipulate the market forces to make them more competitive, and then accept the market's decisions. The first strategy is essentially the public-utility approach, where the monopolist's decisions on price, quality, and rates of return on investment are regulated to approximate competitive market decisions. The second strategy primarily entails making market entry easier, to intensify competition.

Medical care is a complex phenomenon, and recent national strategies for controlling or directing its components have varied. Something of a public-utility approach is developing toward hospitals, for example, on the premise that even in localities where they are not natural monopolies, the best answer usually is not to increase the number or size of inpatient facilities, because undersupply of hospital beds and other inpatient services may not be the basic cause of the upward pressure on prices. With respect to physician services, national initiatives have been directed toward introducing more competition into the markets for MDs and their services. Two major legislative efforts—subsidization of medical education and encouragement of HMOs—were designed in large measure, respectively, (1) to increase the supply and improve the distribution of physicians and (2) to encourage more efficient forms of medical-care organization in the service market, as competitors of the prevailing fee-for-service mode of delivery.[d]

More recently the Federal Trade Commission has entered the health field with new initiatives. In 1974 a Senate subcommittee had held hearings on competition in the health service market,[5] but no additional legislation resulted. Then in 1975 the FTC challenged the AMA's ban on physician advertising and announced that it intended to investigate what appeared to be physician control over Blue Shield organizations.[6] Those moves were followed in the spring of 1976 by an announcement that the FTC was looking into the possibility that

---

[d]Of course, HMOs typically include inpatient as well as outpatient services.

the AMA may have "illegally restrained the supply of physicians and health care services through activities relating to: accreditation of medical schools and graduate programs; definition of fields of practice for physicians and allied personnel; and limitations on forms of health care delivery inconsistent with a traditional fee-for-service approach."[7]

Thus federal attempts have been made to shore up the market mechanism to bring its performance more into line with defined interests of consumers and tax payers. What about professional performance? Here the basic federal strategy has been to articulate some new professional ground rules, to rearrange the incentive structure to induce rather than coerce the desired professional behavior, and to point to the federal option, held in reserve, of replacing profession with government bureau as the decision maker where performance falls short of critical national needs.

The Legislative Milieu

Legislative action on health issues is shaped by a rich configuration of ideological perspectives, economic interests, personality conflicts, the whimsy of chance, and the inherent characteristics of the political process itself. Ideological debate is sometimes real, sometimes forensic, and economic interests are far from monolithic. The professional thrust, for instance, although sometimes unitary, is often fractionated by the way an issue turns with respect to the particularistic interests of subgroups within the medical complex, such as the American Medical Association, the American Hospital Association (AHA), and the Association of American Medical Colleges (AAMC). The AMA's position as spokesman for the profession has declined in recent years. Its membership has fallen to less than half of the nation's physicians, largely older physicians in small, fee-for-service practices. Furthermore, some fissures have opened between the AMA's traditional policies and the immediate interests of the AHA and the AAMC.

The politico-legislative process is complicated also by the fact that the President as well as Congress is responding to changing social needs; and the White House and the legislature are often at odds about the needs and how they should be met. There are tensions between the administrative and legislative bureaucracies. Indeed, there are conflicts within the bureaucracies. Each HEW bureau tends to develop its own programs, its own clientele or constituency among private interest groups, and its own methods of pursuing its goals in the legislative environment. Much of the major health legislation of the last decade has been a compromise of bitterly disparate interests. Often it is the enemies of an act who write its contents and then disclaim responsibility for translating the law's printed pages successfully into the institutional fabric of the health industry. Medicare is a good example. The AMA stringently opposed

Medicare; yet when passage became imminent, it shaped many of its provisions, but accepted no responsibility for the law's successful implementation.

Why would an act be rammed through if the price of success at the enactment level is likely to be failure or mediocrity or stalemate at the effectuation level? Pride in legislative prowess seems to have been a factor in what some advocates saw as premature passage of the HMO law, although in that case, as in others, defenders of the legislative effort reasoned, perhaps correctly, that it was better to put the law onto the books immediately, as the statement of a national sense of direction, even if the tools for implementation were severely restricted. Legislation about medical care may be perceived as reflecting the political realities at any given time. The hesitance, the gingerliness, with which decision making has been moved from profession and market to government reflects not only particularist pressures but also a general skepticism about policy outcomes when attempts are made to increase social control over something as complex, delicately balanced, and internally rationalized as the American medical-care system.

Federal reluctance has been accompanied by ambiguity of direction in the medical field. By brushing aside the question of social control, the Medicare and Medicaid Acts set in motion or exacerbated patterns of institutional behavior that were certain to require further action (e.g., PSRO legislation). The Comprehensive Health Planning (CHP) Act of 1968 was designed to contain a rampant expansion of hospital plant and equipment fed in part by virtually stringless third-party payments, including payments from public funds. The subsequent co-optation of many CHP agencies by hospital and professional interests was partly responsible for the passage of the National Health Planning and Resources Development Act of 1974, which attempted afresh to put planning more firmly into community, rather than professional hands. Sometimes the interlock of legislative measures is forward rather than backward looking, anticipatory rather than corrective. Perhaps those who took a social-reform approach to HMOs, for instance, were more cavalier about the implementation issue than they would have been had not national health insurance seemed imminent at the time.

Quality, Cost Control, and the PSRO

The discussion focuses on Medicare because it has been administered at the federal level, through the Social Security Administration (SSA), rather than shared with the states. Under Medicare, physicians were to be paid their "customary and usual" fees. Hospitals were to be reimbursed at cost. Payments to physicians and hospitals were to be made not directly by the government through SSA but through Blue Shield, Blue Cross, or other insurers acting as the government's fiscal intermediaries, largely because physicians and hospital administrators felt more comfortable dealing with such agents than with the government; that concession, however, placed yet another bureaucratic layer between the taxpayers and the poor, and the "Blues" were generally viewed as sensitive to professional interests.

A noncompetitive supply situation, with costs externalized via third-party payments, is not the climate to foster cost-consciousness among providers or suppliers of services. The only possessor of sufficient market power on the buyer's side, the federal government, declined to use that power to monitor either prices or the manipulation of demand by the sellers. Small wonder that physician incomes ballooned from increased fees,[e] a greater volume of services, and fewer defaults on bills; or that hospital charges, where third-party payment by private insurance as well as by government programs constitutes an even higher percentage of total revenues, rose even more precipitately.

PSRO Origins

The 1972 Social Security Amendments contained a section authorizing the establishment of Professional Standards Review Organizations as a means of reducing overutilization and misutilization under Medicare. Senator Wallace Bennett had proposed PSROs as early as 1970.[8] The PSROs were to be physician groups that would develop and carry out quality and utilization protocols within federal guidelines. The law specifically prohibited the monitoring of physician fees by PSROs. Cost containment was to come through controlling utilization rates, to prevent unnecessary treatment and therefore unnecessary charges to the public purse.

The original Medicare legislation had provided for utilization review by physician staff committees in hospitals and had directed the intermediaries to review claims for abuses. In most cases, however, the review processes were uncoordinated and inadequately motivated. From evidence presented at the hearings on the 1972 Amendments the Senate Committee concluded that review had been largely ineffectual.[9] Whether review under Medicare was being taken seriously by physicians depended more upon whether the hospital could accommodate additional patients than upon the public (and patient) interest in avoiding unnecessary, expensive time spent in confinement.

The PSRO approach purported to give directly to physicians themselves, in approved groupings, the authority to define quality and appropriate utilization,

---

[e]During 1960–65 the average annual rate of increase in physician fees was 2.8 percent; during 1965–70, 6.6 percent. Even though physicians were covered by the general price-control program of the early 1970s, the figure was 5.6 percent during 1970–74. *Basic Charts on Health Care*, prepared by the staff of the Subcommittee on Health, House Committee on Ways and Means, U.S. Government Printing Office, 1975 (WMCP: 94–48), p. 37.

on the principle that "only physicians are, in general, qualified to judge whether services ordered by other physicians are necessary," and also on the premise that the better elements in the profession could be induced to monitor and even discipline the worst, in the public interest. Although the profession had demonstrated some autonomous inclination in that direction—for example, hospital tissue or tumor committees to review surgical procedures postoperatively—the PSRO premise rested more precariously on faith than upon the empirical record.

The ultimate responsibility for establishing PSROs was given to the Secretary of HEW, but he was directed by the law to give first refusal to local medical societies or other professional organizations. To be designated a PSRO, an organization had to be nonprofit, enroll a "substantial portion" of all licensed MDs and DOs (osteopaths) in the designated local area, and not make PSRO membership contingent upon membership in any other professional society (for example, the AMA).[10] The last stipulation, and the fact that the National Professional Standards Review Council (13 physicians) was to be appointed by the Secretary rather than by the AMA and/or other established professional associations, attested the desire of Congress to prevent capture of the PSROs by organized medicine, which had resisted both Medicare and the PSRO idea. The PSRO spear was to be two-pronged, the first aimed at establishing criteria to judge the appropriateness of medical procedures and the second aimed at curtailing hospital admissions, patient bed days, surgery, and other expensive components of care when they are medically unnecessary or inappropriate.

Professional Reaction to PSROs

Organized professional antipathy to the PSRO act was immediate; in fact, some segments of the profession reacted with alarm.[11] The response reflected a widespread physician view of the new law as inherently threatening to the essence of professional prerogative—namely, control over the content of medical practice and over the discipline of profession members. The PSRO issue split the AMA. Advocates of outright repeal overrode more conciliatory voices in the AMA House of Delegates in December 1973,[12] and a series of anti-PSRO materials issued from the headquarters office in succeeding months.[13]

By June 1974, however, the initiative had been seized by House of Delegates members who regarded peer review as an idea whose time had come and who wished to make sure that peer review was lodged securely in physician hands. Under the law, the HEW Secretary was directed to establish PSROs in locales where physician initiative was still absent on January 1, 1976. Mindful of that alternative, Dr. Claude E. Welch, chairman of an AMA Task Force on Guidelines of Care, cautioned physicians to "move rapidly enough so that the government will never find it necessary to give the (PSRO) implementation to state departments of health, a move that would tend to divide the profession deeply, or to medical schools, which are totally unprepared to meet the challenge."[14]

Going on to predict that review of professional practice would surely increase anyway, Dr. Welch asked whether the medical profession would "sit behind the table in cooperation with the government, which serves as the representative of the public, or . . . stand on the carpet to be judged by others."[15]

The strategy of the conciliatory group within the AMA leadership was to try for amendments in the PSRO guidelines rather than for repeal. Since the fall of 1973 the AMA had been negotiating with HEW for a contract to develop "screening criteria" for use by PSROs. The negotiations cooled after the House of Delegates' hostile action in December had caused Senator Bennett and other PSRO supporters to ask why federal funds for implementing the law should be given to those so pungently opposed to it.[16] When the House of Delegates reversed the December action at its June 1974 meeting in Chicago, a contract for a million dollars was quickly let to the AMA, with subcontracts to the major medical specialty groups, to produce model sets of criteria to cover diagnosis and treatment procedures for up to 75 percent of short-stay hospital admissions.[17] Those criteria sets were to be offered to hospital committees at the local PSRO level for adoption, amendment, or whatever, since the hospital committees were to make the final decisions about medical-appropriateness criteria.

New tensions soon developed, however, between HEW and the AMA over utilization review (UR). The Secretary issued UR regulations for Medicare and Medicaid patients on November 29, 1974, to take effect on February 1, 1975, but the date was later changed to July 1. On February 20 the AMA filed suit in a Chicago federal district court, and on May 27 the court enjoined the regulations, an action sustained by an appellate court on July 22. In September HEW announced its intention to revise the regulations. A new set, in tentative form that allowed 60 days for comment, was finally published in late March 1976.[f] In the interim, the AMA and HEW had worked out compromises in particularly sensitive areas.

Two such areas concerned review of hospital admissions for Medicaid and Medicare and the role of nonphysician personnel in the Medicare review process.[g] The old HEW regulations, announced in November 1974, had required 100 percent review of hospital admissions, within one working day, and the inclusion of other professionals, such as optometrists, pharmacists, and nurses, in the UR procedures. The AMA's counterproposal included the following: that across-the-board review be limited to physicians with a "demonstrable history of over-utilization" and to "those medical conditions and procedures which the local

[f]*Federal Register* for March 30, 1976 contains the new set and gives the background materials used here. Although some states have resisted including Medicaid under PSROs, it seems clear that Congress intended such inclusions and many PSROs already are monitoring Medicaid as well as Medicare services.

[g]See *Statement of the American Medical Association Regarding Utilization Review Regulations of the Department of Health, Education, and Welfare*, August 29, 1975 (processed) for the range of AMA objections. The two mentioned here were the subject of the injunction.

utilization review committee determines are frequently overutilized"; that, otherwise, review of admissions be done by sampling, "within a reasonable time," and by "duly licensed physicians" only; and that in doubtful cases, great weight be given to the judgment of the attending or admitting physician.

The highlights of the proposed new PSRO regulations, issued after the negotiations, may be summarized as follows: The medical staff of a hospital to which the local PSRO has delegated UR responsibility must designate at least two physicians as the UR committee, which can also include nonphysician personnel *at the medical staff's discretion.* Whether on the committee or not, nonphysician health professionals must be consulted by the committee when their experience and knowledge would be helpful. Review of all admissions must be completed within three working days. Two categories of review criteria must be developed by the hospital medical staff. The first relates to diagnoses or medical conditions that in themselves require admission; the second relate to conditions that require further screening. The UR committee may delegate to a nonphysician, say a nurse, the determination of whether an admission meets the criteria of the first category. If it does not, a physician member of the UR committee will review the case with reference to the criteria of the second category. If the reviewer determines that the admitting physician was correct, the issue is settled; but it takes two UR committee members, after consulting the admitting physician, to make a nonnecessity ruling stick.[18]

Quick review of admissions is critical for cost control. Although a quality review (medical audit) may be done retrospectively, it is essential that the determination of nonnecessity in such a costly item as hospitalization be made prospectively if possible, or very promptly if it is not feasible to screen before admission. Surgery is another case where prospective review is essential for successful cost control.

Costs and Professional Responsibility

Although by February 1976 it was estimated that one-third of the nation was already covered by PSROs actually carrying out review of medical care and that another third had PSROs moving toward operational status,[19] the experience with PSROs is still new, and the information available contains mixed signals. One reservation often expresses concern whether the cost savings from curtailing unnecessary services will be greater than the administrative costs of the PSRO review processes. At one recent congressional hearing the medical director of the Colorado statewide PSRO cited savings of $6,400,000 from curtailment of patient-days for Medicare and Medicaid patients, as compared with a program expenditure of only $1,500,000—a ratio of roughly one to four.[20] Whereas heartened by that report, HEW officials in Washington have repeatedly warned against overoptimism; moreover, spokesmen often have deemphasized the cost-control aspects of the PSRO program. Thus the acting head of the Health Services Administration, at that same hearing, stated:

While PSROs have been viewed by many as primarily a mechanism of cost control and only secondarily a means of quality assurance, early implementation of the program indicates that PSROs most effectively function as a quality assurance mechanism which can achieve cost savings through decreasing unnecessary or inappropriate services, including unnecessary surgery.[21]

The Senate Finance Committee, however, in advocating the Social Security Amendments of 1972, had projected that "the PSRO provision, properly implemented, should result in substantial reductions" in Medicare and Medicaid costs.[22] Of course, the cost implications of the PSRO program are not all downward. To the degree that quality audit discovers underutilization, or inappropriate procedures that should be replaced by procedures that can be obtained only at higher prices, PSROs could raise the costs of care. Whether the net effect of PSROs will be cost curtailing or cost elevating depends on many variables to which even preliminary numbers cannot yet be assigned.

The health systems agencies (HSAs), created by the National Health Planning and Resources Development Act of 1974, are replacing the CHP agencies as local instruments of assessing needs and monitoring resource uses, particularly with respect to inpatient facilities. Because need assessment is closely related to questions of quality and use, the success of the HSAs in preventing overexpansion of hospital beds and equipment in their locales will depend in part on access to data developed by the PSROs. There is likely to be tension, however, between community-oriented HSAs and physician-dominated PSROs. For example, there is the issue of the confidentiality of PSRO data—information from individual physician-performance profiles and review-committee records as well as from patient medical charts. There is also the fact that patient, consumer, and citizen interests are not always neatly consonant or mutually coextensive, particularly in the area of costs. The physician ethic is patient oriented; the HSAs are by design more concerned with the interests of consumers and taxpayers. An interesting question raised by the PSROs is whether MDs can play—indeed, ought to try to play—the double role of patient advocate and cost controller; the roles can be conflicting.

The second contingency is the degree to which PSRO physicians will accept responsibility commensurate with their authority. Here again, experience thus far is mixed. In some locales, where enough members of the profession either approve of PSROs or have accepted peer review as inevitable and are trying to make physician control of PSROs work, PSROs are reported to be functioning effectively. Appraisals of other situations are less optimistic. Dr. Robert H. Barnes head of a nonprofit corporation financed by the Washington State Medical Association to help community hospitals develop review programs suggested:

Most physicians feel harassed and oppressed by the federal government and would like to get away from it. Even though thousands of physicians have signed up [for PSRO], the real support may be quite shallow and superficial. Some tell me the support is justified only because of the lack of an alternative, or for fear of alternatives.[23]

PSROs and the Consumer

The role that consumer interests should play in PSROs is an important and potentially cost-sensitive issue. Two aspects of the issue are discussed here: consumer voice in policy formation and consumer participation in the review process. The board of directors of a PSRO is elected by the PSRO's physician membership. In some localities one or more nonphysicians have been chosen to speak for consumers. Perhaps the greatest tension thus far between consumer spokesmen and physicians on the boards has concerned consumer access to the individual physician profiles developed by the PSRO review committees, at public expense. Some consumer representatives have argued that those profiles, showing which physicians have poor records, should be made public. After all, for a market to function competitively, consumer choice must be informed by knowledge about the options. But there has been strong physician resistance to such disclosure. Also, developing a vigorous consumer input into PSRO policy is difficult, for in order to serve on the PSRO board, consumer representatives must be elected (and reelected) by the PSRO's physician membership, rather than by a consumer constituency whom they are presumed to represent.

Why are PSRO boards (and HEW) so reluctant to release the records of physicians who persistently ignore or contravene the quality and utilization guidelines? A staff member of one of the earliest PSROs said recently, "The PSROs are just getting established, and, let's face it, we aren't going anywhere without physician support. Confidentiality is an explosive issue." A staff person in another PSRO stated, "We believe a more effective approach is to handle the problem internally, at least at first—to try to re-educate offenders rather than threaten them with exposure."[24] Incidentally, because PSROs are directed only at medical bills paid from public revenues, it is perhaps the citizen-taxpayer interests rather than consumer interests that should be included in PSRO policy-making. Still, other congressional action has portrayed a substantial commitment to making the market function more effectively, and it is against that backdrop that federal hesitance about disclosure of physician profiles must be evaluated.[h]

Consumer (or citizen) input into the quality and utilization-review process

---

[h]As HEW policy now stands, not even Medicare representatives are to have access to physician or institution profiles; moreover, efficiencies developed by one *PSRO* can not be used as a lever on *PSRO* in other locales.

itself, as opposed to participation in general policy formation, is an issue that has scarcely been raised, even by consumer groups themselves. From the public-interest viewpoint, the only acceptable rationale for assigning to the medical profession the development and application of quality criteria is not that physicians have a professional right to the assignment but that they and only they are competent to fulfill it. But is that so?

Dr. Barnes's reservations, mentioned above, go primarily to the *application* of quality criteria, once they are determined, at the local level, where physician leaders understand the issues but practicing physicians do not. Dr. Barnes suggested that physicians do not wish to review other physicians, and may fail to change poor practices because of mediocre reviews.[25]

But what about physician *determination,* as opposed to *application,* of quality criteria? There are no objective measures of medical-care quality. Promising methods of linking medical procedures to outcomes in patient-health status are in their infancy, when they have appeared at all. What criteria the PSRO committee can develop, in the present state of the art, are at best normative statements of what physicians—the best physicians? the average physicians?—are doing, or what the present doctrine is. This circumstance raises the question of whether "appropriate" or "medically necessary" procedures should be defined at the most advanced level of medical technology or at some minimally acceptable level of quality assurance. The cost implications of that choice are apparent. So are the moral implications, and here as in other aspects of the quality issue, it is not at all clear that the *choice between* the minimal and optimal standards should be made by physicians, even if one concedes that physicians should *define* those two standards.

Another complication of the quality issue relates to this question: should quality be defined solely in technical dimensions? Very little in the PSRO initiative suggests an alternative approach to definition; yet surely consumer satisfaction and convenience are important dimensions of quality. Although objections to those dimensions stress their immeasurability, measurement in their case poses no greater difficulty—perhaps less—than in the case of technical competence. Including patient satisfaction and convenience would have implications for both costs and the proper locus of decision. Changing outpatient schedules to reduce patient waiting time, or revamping hospital routines to serve patient rather than nurse and doctor convenience, could increase the cost of providing care, and hence prices and costs for consumers and taxpayers. That approach might be counterproductive as calculated in rationales internal to medical delivery systems, which tend to value the patient's time at zero and the doctor's time at infinity, but in the larger socioeconomic context, the cost increase might be offset to the degree that time formerly spent by patients in waiting rooms could be transferred to more productive activities.

Including patient satisfaction and convenience in the quality calculus might be unattractive to physicians because they have no special competence for measuring those dimensions—indeed, the physician's training, experience, and professional ideology may incapacitate him or her in that sphere, so development and application of criteria that include satisfaction and convenience might require that PSRO quality committees include, in addition to patients themselves, social scientists skilled in measuring patient responses to alternate modes of medical treatment and alternate modes of arranging medical care. The result would be further dilution of professional control over quality assurance.

Why not require the same kind of quality and efficiency review for all patients rather than merely for the old and the poor? By confining its quality-assurance and utilization-review initiative to Medicare and Medicaid patients, the federal government in effect has elected to use its force in a limited economic role, acting as a *monopsonist*, that is, as a possessor of monopoly on the buyer's side of the market for medical services. In other words, the government is (1) protecting the interests of citizens who as a collectivity of taxpayers purchase medical care for selected groups, rather than (2) assuming the role of a political instrument for citizens who as consumers must purchase medical care severally for themselves. Extending PSRO activity to all patients, or even making the present PSRO findings on physician performance available to the general public, might have a cost-containing effect on all medical bills. But to take that action Congress would have to make a far less ambiguous commitment to regulating quality and strengthening competition in the market than it as yet has seemed willing to do.

Medical Subsidies: Efforts to Increase
Physician Supply and Distribution

Growing public concern in the late 1950s and 1960s about an actual or potential "doctor shortage" prompted the establishment of a series of ad hoc national commissions. The commissions' reports pointed with alarm to the failure of physicians' numbers even to keep pace with population growth;[26] moreover, it became apparent that the situation was not likely to be remedied without federal subsidization of expanded medical school facilities.

The Coming of Federal Subsidies

Federal contributions to medical-education centers had been confined largely to research grants, with the burgeoning National Institutes of Health channeling large sums to medical-school faculties in the 1950s. In 1963, the Health Professions Education Assistance Act (HPEA)[i] made construction grants available

---

[i]Although the HPEA and other acts discussed in this section were not confined to physicians, only those provisions relating to physicians' education are discussed here, because of this chapter's focus on MDs.

and also provided funds for student loans. Those two moves attempted to tie federal aid more closely to increased enrollments, which eventually would produce an increase in physician supply. Two years later, in amending the act, Congress deepened its commitment to medical schools by providing funds for certain kinds of operational costs, particularly improvements in the quality of faculty and curricula. Again, aid was made contingent upon agreements to expand enrollment.

The adequacy of these programs was brought into question by several new surveys, the most important done in 1967 by the National Advisory Commission on Health Manpower.[27] The demand for medical services had trended upward in the 1950s and early 1960s under the stimulus of population increases, shifts toward an older population, rising incomes and educational levels, and great advances in the biomedical sciences. Medicare and Medicaid brought a new upward jolt to demand. Those developments, together with the financial stress of medical schools, dictated the assumption by the federal government of major, long-term responsibility for the survival and expansion of high-quality medical education, a responsibility that traditionally had been borne primarily by the states and private philanthropy.

Congressional acts of 1968 and 1970[28] addressed the worsening position of the medical schools, beset by inflation and the race to keep their equipment current with proliferating medical technologies. It was not until the Comprehensive Health Manpower Training Act of 1971, however, that federal subsidization shifted from an essentially ad hoc, situational approach to a more orderly, ongoing commitment that permitted the schools to engage in long-term planning within a context of relative financial security. A Carnegie Commission report[29] on health manpower earlier that year had made an impact on members of Congress by calling into question the relative health status of Americans, as compared with the citizens of other Western nations, and by linking the invidious comparison not only to a shortage of physicians but also to their maldistribution.

In the 1971 act the principal method selected for underwriting the stability of medical colleges was capitation grants to medical schools. That strategy tightened the bonds between federal assistance and enrollment because thenceforth the main subsidies would be distributed among schools on the basis of student counts. The 1971 act is still the primary health manpower law, its various authorities having been extended beyond its original expiration date of June 30, 1974 when Congress failed to agree on a replacement bill. In addition to basic capitation grants, determined by the number of students and graduates, the law offered bonuses for three-year (as opposed to four-year) curricula, for training physicians' assistants, and for an enrollment increase larger than the minimum increase required to participate in the capitation-grant program. Even greater institutional support may be given where it is warranted by heavy start-up costs or other special needs.

Loans and scholarships up to $3,500 per year have been made to students studying in the United States or abroad, and there are special scholarships or loan-forgiveness options for graduates who practice in underserved areas. Assistance for construction of new public or nonprofit private-school facilities include grants-in-aid of up to 80 percent of the costs; loan guarantees and interest subsidies are also available for nonprofit schools. The 1971 legislation and subsequent extensions of it also provide funds for a series of special programs designed to serve specific national policy priorities, such as shifting more graduate medical education into the primary-care specialties, raising the percentage of women and minority groups in medical-student bodies, increasing physician productivity by developing new kinds of auxiliary personnel, and moving more educational resources into rural areas. Medical schools receiving capitation funds have been expected to participate in at least three of nine special programs.[j]

As a result of the new capitation approach, medical schools did gain financial stability, but at a price. What had turned out to be, in effect, relatively stringless federal funds prior to 1971 were from that time on to be more specifically contingent upon a school's affirmatively addressing a set of national needs defined not by the schools or even by the profession but by the larger society through its political institutions. Those priorities included not only an increase in the supply of physicians but an improvement in their spatial distribution and specialty mix.

Subsidies, Numbers, and Distribution

How effective has the new approach been? Given the long lead time necessary to produce physicians, five years is too short a time to measure the efficacy of the legislative initiatives. The congressional committees responsible for health manpower legislation—the Committee on Interstate and Foreign Commerce in the House and the Committee on Labor and Public Welfare in the Senate—have attempted to assess the programs' results in a series of hearings and reports during 1974-76, when unsuccessful attempts were being made to pass a new law. At this writing, bills passed respectively by the House in 1975 and by the Senate in 1976 are in the conference process. The two committee reports[30] contain summaries of previous laws, evaluations of their impact, and a rationale for the respective bills the reports accompany. The two committees are clearly in conflict on a number of issues, including (1) *where* and *which specialties* physicians should practice, and (2) *how the determination should be made.*

---

[j]Report by the Committee on Interstate and Foreign Commerce, U.S. House of Representatives, 94th Congress, 1st Session, June 7, 1975 (Report No. 94-266, to accompany H.R. 5546, a health manpower bill). This volume has a good brief summary of previous health manpower legislation as well as a detailed discussion of the proposed law.

It seems clear that the incentives, guidelines, and sanctions contained in the 1971 act, and in its immediate predecessors, have been effective in raising the numbers of students who have exited from or are now moving through the medical-school pipelines. In 1963-64 fewer than 8,800 first-year medical students were enrolled in American Medical Schools. By 1973-74 that figure had risen to over 14,000.[31] First-year classes have grown at an annual rate of 6.6 percent since 1965, as compared with 1.3 percent for the preceding 15 years. It has been estimated that current enrollment will produce more than 16,000 graduates in 1979, 78 percent more than the 1971 graduating class.[32]

Is enrollment now high enough? The answer depends not only upon how the graduates will be distributed spatially and the percentage going into primary-care specialties but also upon the way medical care is organized and paid for—and many other variables such as the hours MDs are willing to work, and their productivity. There is no set of objective criteria from which the "proper" number and distribution of physicians can be neatly derived. Yet there is a substantial consensus that the existing spatial distribution is inequitable, especially where communities without physicians, or with physician-population ratios much lower than average, contribute their share of the state and federal taxes that so heavily subsidize the education of MDs.

Spatial Maldistribution

Inequalities in the geographical distribution of physicians have been documented in many studies.[33] The essentially rural state of South Dakota, for example, has one doctor per 1,316 persons, whereas New York state has one doctor per 500 or fewer. Within metropolitan areas physicians have moved to the suburbs, leaving many inner-city residents without adequate access to medical care. In the Chicago area, for example, a shift of physicians from the city itself to the more affluent surrounding areas between 1950 and 1970 resulted in a gain of 130 percent for the suburbs and a loss of 35 percent for the city.[34]

Confronting the apparent inability or disinclination of the existing market forces, or the professional ethic as currently practiced, to redress the spatial maldistribution, the federal government has developed several strategies to remedy the situation. One strategy—the Area Health Education Center (AHEC)— was directed at the capitation funds given to medical schools; the other—loan forgiveness for service in underserved areas—was directed at subsidies channeled to students themselves.

The AHEC strategy was included in the 1971 act. An AHEC is a clinical-teaching center developed in an outlying community hospital by a medical school, in association with other professional schools. AHECs serve several purposes. They upgrade the quality and quantity of local health care by establishing medical residencies, with appropriate supportive services for instruction and medical-care delivery in areas that lie beyond the usual medical school constellations, and by providing continuing education for doctors already practicing there. Furthermore, it was conjectured that some of the residents trained in such settings might build the kind of attachments that would cause them to stay on after their training period had ended. Establishing AHECs is one of the options medical schools can choose as a quid pro quo for continued federal support under the capitation program; in fact, the bills reported out of the House and Senate Committees in 1975 and 1976, respectively, would increase AHEC appropriations. The bills also provide funds for exposing more medical-school undergraduates to underserved areas by arranging part of their clinical training in such locales.

Concern for the public welfare also inhabited medical colleges,[k] where a growing minority of distinguished medical educators articulated their unease about a widening gap between the highly "technologized," highly specialized, hospital-based medicine taught in the front-running medical school complexes and outpatient-oriented practices in the hinterlands. How to put advancing medical knowledge about cardiovascular disease and other major killers at the service of the great bulk of American citizens was one challenge, and the reach of a service-oriented medical elite is perhaps best illustrated by the provocative report of the DeBakey commission appointed by President Johnson in 1964. Directed to recommend strategies for bringing heart disease, cancer, and stroke under better control and treatment, the commission proposed webs of patient-care delivery, radiating from centers of medical education and research in an integrated national health system whose financial stability would be under-written by the federal government.

The thrust of the concept was blunted by federal funds competition from Medicare and Medicaid—and the Vietnam war— and also by opposition from organized medicine, which, like the business community and congressional conservatives, saw in the scheme the socialization of health care. Very little of the DeBakey plan found its way into the Regional Medical Programs (RMP) act of 1966, which, the sponsoring House committee emphasized, "is intended to be administered in such a way as to make no change whatsoever in the traditional methods of furnishing medical care to patients in the United States, or to financing such care."[l] The AHECs are a modest initiative compared with the DeBakey plan or even with the RMP; AHECs, like the RMP, entail no basic challenge to existing delivery arrangements, and their scale and scope are even narrower.

---

[k]And other institutions in the private sector, but this exposition, as stated earlier, is concerned primarily with physicians.

[l]For a spritely description of the role played by the AMA in defeating the DeBakey Plan, see Barbara and John Ehrenreich, *The American Health Empire: Power, Profits, and Politics* (New York: Random House, 1971), Chapter XV.

A more direct approach to moving well-trained physicians into medically needy geographical areas is contained in the plans to permit physicians to "pay off" federal student loans by service in ghettos and hinterlands. The debate that loan-forgiveness proposals have evoked is part of the much larger, deeply controversial issue concerning the degree to which physicians should bear the financial burden of their medical education. A strict market approach would place the full cost of medical training upon the student, who, under a policy of open admissions to medical school, would decide to make or not to make the required investment of his own or borrowed funds after weighing, along with other considerations, the expected return on the investment from future career earnings. Even physicians preferring to practice in the suburbs might spill over into the inner cities and the rural areas if price competition from an eventual oversupply of doctors in the suburbs made practice elsewhere more attractive. In the long run that approach might greatly reduce federal outlays, or at least shift federal funds from the training level to the delivery level if patient purchase of medical services in the central city and the rural areas were more heavily subsidized.[m]

No measure under serious consideration in Congress goes to that extreme. One reason is an uncertainty about the independence of supply and demand in the medical field. Some observers have suggested that the demand for medical care may increase as the supply of physicians grows, because physicians, who control the demand for medical services to a substantial degree, will intensify services per patient if the number of patients per physician declines through competition from greater physician numbers. To the degree that that is true, increasing the physician supply would, in addition to servicing a rising demand for care, ipso facto increase that demand, which might reach unacceptable proportions under a policy of open-ended supply as discussed above.

Subsidies for Schools or Students?

Recent proposals from the executive and legislative branches of the federal government that medical students should pay a larger share of their educational costs stem both from a deepening ethical sensitivity about the taxes of the poor contributing to high-income careers and from a desire to use the medical student's increased financial burden as a lever to move more graduates into underserved areas. How much do four years of medical school cost? Because estimating the cost of producing a graduate is complicated by the difficulty

---

[m]For a market-oriented study that questions the need for federal subsidies to assure adequate numbers of physicians, see C.T. Stewart and C.M. Sidayao, *Increasing the Supply of Medical Personnel*, (Washington D.C.: American Enterprise Institute for Public Policy Research, March 1973).

of separating costs for instruction, for research, and for the medical services that medical schools provide as part of the educational complex, no adequate data were available when the 1971 act was in preparation. The act therefore directed that costs be studied, and the Institute of Medicine of the National Academy of Sciences made a study for the academic year of 1972-73. Average net educational expenditures per student per year were estimated to be about $9,700.[n] The capitation program has covered about 20 percent of that figure, with other federal funds, state funds, endowments, and tuition payments contributing to the remainder.

When the House Subcommittee held its 1974 hearings on new health manpower legislation, the Nixon administration's position, which had considerable support in Congress, was that the cost of a medical education ought to be borne primarily by its recipient, either concurrently or from the substantial income the medical graduate usually enjoys once he becomes established in practice. One proposal before the subcommittee was to replace the capitation subsidies with increases in tuition, accompanied by an expanded student-loan program. The burden of repaying the loans almost certainly would boost applications to the National Health Service Corps, which had been established in 1972.[35] to provide MDs and other health professionals for communities where medical services were critically undersupplied.

Eliminating the capitation program entirely would shorten the federal wrench upon medical school policies; to the degree that subsidies were shifted from the schools to students, it would become more difficult to influence or shape institutional behavior toward national purposes and priorities. An interesting question for the law makers: whose behavior was it more important to influence—the medical school's or the graduate's—in trying to effectuate federal policies? The bill that eventually emerged from the House Committee in mid-1975 placed a foot on each strategic path. It retained capitation funding, but it made the capitation subsidy a draft upon graduating students' future incomes or services. In taking that approach the committee was influenced by the fact that federal subsidies had become more generous for students in health-professional schools (including medical colleges) than for students in other educational programs. According to the committee report, professional schools in the health field are

the only schools in the United States which receive direct, unencumbered Federal subsidies in support of educational activities. Such support represents 7 percent of the total income of such schools and at least 20 percent of the cost of educating

---

[n]Data from the IOM study are cited in the House Committee Report 16-18. The figure of $9,700 was derived by subtracting from total education costs of $14,100 the offsetting revenues of $2,100 and $1,300 for research and patient-care, respectively, which are attributable to services performed by medical students.

their students. In contrast, *tuition* payments represent ten percent of total revenues of health profession schools while, according to a recent survey of 90 state and land-grant universities, tuition payments contribute 14.2 percent of the revenues of such institutions.[36]

In other words, students in health-professional schools were bearing, through tuition payments, a relatively small portion of their training costs.

The loan-forgiveness program contained in the HPEA of 1965 authorized cancellation of federal student loans of up to 50 percent (plus interest), at 10 percent per year, for practice in a certified health manpower-shortage area and up to 100 percent, at 15 percent per year, if the certified locale was designated additionally to be a rural low-income area. The figures were upgraded by the 1971 act. The program as amended applied to student loans from any source and provided forgiveness of federal loans (and repayment by HEW of nonfederal loans) up to 85 percent rather than 50 percent for practice in a shortage area— 60 percent for the first two years and 25 percent for the third year.

The House committee report pointed to 405 physicians, dentists, and other health professionals having been placed in 196 underserved communities in 40 states by 1975. The Senate committee report cited two less encouraging studies. One by the General Accounting Office (GAO) and the other by an independent research organization under a HEW contract showed that these entirely voluntary programs had been "unsuccessful."[39] The GAO found that of 30,000 medical and dental students who had received loans between 1965 and 1972, only 86 physicians and 133 dentists had had a portion of their loans cancelled by October, 1973. Both studies questioned the effectiveness of loan forgiveness as an incentive even for the fewer than 1 percent of graduates taking advantage of it, because most of them appeared to have located in shortage areas for other reasons.

The Senate committee bill retains the student-loan program but provides for its phase-out in 1980. The bill greatly expands the National Health Service Corps scholarship program. Scholarships are available for two to four years and cover tuition and other educational costs plus a stipend for living expenses. The recipient signs a contract to join the corps upon graduation and to serve the same number of years for which he received scholarships. Moreover, the bill specifies that in return for continuing capitation aid, medical schools collectively must reserve at least 25 percent of their upcoming first-year enrollment slots for students who have agreed to receive corps scholarships. If that figure is not met voluntarily by the schools on a national level during the first year after the bill becomes law, each school must reserve 30 percent of its first-year places the following year. The figure for the third year is 35 percent. Giving students corps scholarships in advance is a more direct and probably more cost-efficient approach than the retrospective loan-cancellation program.

The Senate committee report points to the original use of capitation subsidies to induce medical schools to increase their enrollment.

Now the Committee believes that the expansion of the medical schools' class size has been sufficient to provide the Nation an adequate number of physicians if they are properly distributed by geographic area and by specialty.[38]

Thus the Senate committee bill would retain the capitation rate and use it as a lever to achieve *distribution* rather than *size* goals in the supply of physicians.

At the hearings on the House committee bill, representatives of the Association of American Medical Colleges had strongly opposed proposals to eliminate capitation subsidies. Moreover, the AAMC spokesman perceived increased tuition charges to replace capitation payments as unacceptable:

Nearly all medical students would need financial assistance to meet the higher tuition expected under the proposal, and most of them would seek aid through a National Health Service Corps Scholarship, with its mandatory service obligation. Such a system comes perilously close to being involuntary national service imposed in a highly discriminatory way on a single group of citizens. The constitutionality of such a system seems open to challenge.[o]

When the Senate committee proposed to keep the capitation program but to link it mandatorily to expansion of the National Health Service Corps, the AAMC argued that generous corps scholarships would attract enough students without encumbering the medical schools with quotas, and that if a percentage figure were set, it ought to apply to a national goal rather than to individual schools.[39] As a concession, the Senate bill gives the schools a year to comply collectively on a voluntary basis; the bill goes on, however, to provide for mandatory compliance if voluntarism fails. This approach by the Senate committee is another indication of a growing reluctance either to permit the profession to determine national priorities or to count on the profession to discipline the behavior of its members (whether individuals or institutions) toward compliance with a national priority.

This is not to suggest that the Congress is insensitive to professional interests, even to the economic interests of individual physicians. The eligibility of a community for a corps physician is determined by criteria developed by HEW. In the House committee bill, communities applying for designation as shortage areas must submit statements from their state or local professional societies, as well as from local government, that additional health professionals are needed— this, in spite of the fact that a definition of "underserved" might rest in many instances on relatively objective criteria whose application is not necessarily

---

[o]*Hearings* on Health Manpower and Nurse Training, Subcommittee on Public Health and Environment, House Committee on Interstate and Foreign Commerce, 93rd Congress, 2nd Session. May and June, 1974, I, 836-7. The administration's position was reiterated in a letter addressed to the committee by the Secretary of HEW, which is included in the committee report, pp. 78-79.

facilitated (indeed, it may be impeded) by professional training, experience, and particularist interests. The Senate bill merely requires the Secretary to take comments from professional groups into account, along with many other considerations such as doctor-population ratios, health status indicator rates, percentages of foreign medical graduates practicing in the locale, and the recommendations of official health-planning agencies.

Specialty Maldistribution

The other kind of maldistribution that congressional initiatives have addressed concerns the division of physicians among the medical specialties, particularly the percentage of doctors in primary care. In 1949, 50 percent of all physicians looked upon themselves as general practitioners, or nonspecialists. That figure had dropped to 16 percent by 1974. Physician specialists increased from 37 percent to 80 percent in the same period. Specialization, which typically entails about three years of training beyond medical school graduation, is usually acquired through residencies established in hospitals. The relation of such hospitals to medical-school complexes may range from direct to quite casual. The number of residencies increased 70 percent between 1950 and 1960 and another 44 percent in the next decade, to a total of 46,000 by 1970. In 1975 the figure was 54,000.

The Senate committee report referred to studies that estimated up to 85 percent of all health problems can be managed by primary-care providers: general practitioners or specialists in family practice, general internal medicine, general pediatrics, and obstetrics and gynecology. It is resource-wasteful and cost-inefficient to have noncomplex, routine care provided by physicians trained to handle secondary and tertiary health problems. Yet the percentage of physicians in primary-care specialties declined from about 71 percent in 1949 to 44 percent in 1970. Moreover, by the academic year of 1973-74, only 39 percent of physicians in such training programs were enrolled in the primary-care specialties. The reason was not a scarcity of residencies in the primary-care area; of the 1,210 family-practice and general-practice residencies offered in 1970, only 43 percent were filled, the lowest percentage for an approved residency program for any specialty. General surgery, for example, filled 91 percent of its vacancies. The committee's immediate goal was 50 percent of the new crop of physicians in primary-care specialties—57 percent counting Ob-Gyns.

A startling statistic is 1.7 residency openings for every medical-school graduate in 1974. Residencies have continued to proliferate—almost doubling between 1965 and 1975—for a variety of reasons, including the explosion of biomedical knowledge, the higher incomes enjoyed by specialists, and the prestige of the residency, for both the school and the hospital. Moreover, residents are relatively inexpensive inputs into research, teaching, and patient-care programs—about $12,000 for a resident as compared with $55,000 for a fully trained physician.

Because hospitals concentrate on inpatient care, residencies emphasize inpatient rather than outpatient training. Also, it is easier for hospitals to support residents' services in inpatient care because of the cost-reimbursement policies of Medicare, Blue Cross, and other third-party payers; the inpatient services given by residents can be included in the per-diem charge. There are over 4,000 of these residency programs in the nation, accredited by review committees sponsored by the national specialty boards and the AMA.[p] The result has been an expansion of first-year residency positions far beyond the number of students exiting from American medical schools. Excess positions have been filled increasingly by graduates of foreign medical colleges (FMGs)— mostly foreigners but some Americans—with many of the foreigners settling in the United States under the liberalized immigration laws of 1965. Because of relatively low scores by FMGs on qualifying exams and the intrusion of language and cultural differences into patient care, public concern over threats to quality have surfaced, and the House committee bill proposes to ameliorate the problem by restricting the number of first-year residencies to 125 percent of the American medical schools' graduating students by 1980.

In addition to reducing the *total number* of residencies, the House bill proposes to review the *distribution* of residencies among the medical specialties for the purpose of bringing numbers more closely into line with the best estimates of future needs. At the time the bill cleared the committee in mid-1975, the Institute of Medicine (IOM) already was engaged in a project, mandated by Congress in its 1973 amendments to the Social Security Act, to study the extent to which Medicare and Medicaid funds were supporting an excess supply of medical specialists (as discussed above) and to recommend ways in which such funds could be used to support a more rational distribution of physician manpower both geographically and by specialty.[q] The IOM researchers, like others, were unable to identify a group of objective criteria for designing a specialty distribution that would serve the best interests of the nation even in 1975, let alone in 1985 or 1990—and yet the lead time necessary to plan the production of specialists can easily stretch to 10 or 15 years.

Specialty Mix: Who Should Decide?

Who should decide the specialty distribution; which is to say, who should determine the number and kinds of residencies available to medical graduates?

---

[p]This whole discussion of specialty maldistribution relies heavily upon the Senate and House reports. The quotation is from the former, at 203.

[q]The author's respect for the complexities of determining a "rational" distribution by specialty was deepened by service on an advisory panel of the IOM study.

That question has become one of the most controversial issues in the congressional arena. The House committee bill gives primary authority to profession. Although, in certifying residencies, the specialty boards traditionally had concerned themselves almost exclusively with quality, the boards, together with other professional groups, began in 1972 to tackle the problem of distribution. Five professional organizations—the AMA, the AAMC, the American Hospital Association, the Council of Medical Specialty Societies, and the American Board of Medical Specialties—had formed two consortiums: the Coordinating Council on Medical Education (CCME) and the Liaison Committee on Graduate Medical Education (LCGME). The LCGME has primary responsibility in the accreditation field; one CCME task is to oversee the policy implications of LCGME's activities, and it was stipulated that major policies affecting graduate education must have the approval of all five of the parental organizations.

It was the House committee's opinion that:

The formation of these two committees—representing the vast majority of the professional and physical resources related to medical education—constitutes a recognition of the responsibility to influence graduate medical education so that it will be responsive to societal needs. These committees have the potential, if afforded the authority, to integrate this responsibility into the development of a uniform policy which can meet the needs of the public by controlling the production of adequate numbers of well qualified specialists, with appropriate emphasis on the most needed specialties and the geographic location of the site of training.[40]

The committee's bill directs the Secretary of HEW to accept an application from the LCGME "to become the sole agency responsible for the review and accreditation of each medical residency program in the United States." The CCME would be given first refusal of the task of deciding how many residencies in each specialty will be established in the United States in future years. Thus the committee "has made every effort short of mandating it" to ensure that these two professionally based organizations would preside over the nation's efforts to redress specialty maldistribution.

Within the CCME, AMA representatives soon announced that the association would not participate in setting quotas for specialties. At the House committee hearings in 1974 both the AMA and the AAMC had disagreed with the committee's approach. The AAMC representatives appeared to prefer the approach. The AAMC representatives appeared to prefer the approach taken in the 1973 Social Security amendments and pointed to the IOM study already in progress.[41] The AMA objected to using an elevation of accreditation standards to control entry into the specialties and argued that, instead, the way to recruit more young doctors into primary care was to make it more attractive.

The 1971 act had inaugurated a special-project grant program for "family-medicine" residencies, and by 1975 over 200 programs had been approved. Moreover, the American Board of Family Practice, which was organized medicine's twentieth recognized specialty, already had certified 5,800 practicing physicians. An AMA representative at the 1974 hearings pointed to the success of the family-practice residency programs in attracting medical-school graduates and reiterated the AMA goal of having at least 50 percent of the nation's graduating physicians enter advanced training in primary care.

Spokesmen for the American Board of Medical Specialties and other groups referred to activities already in process under professional initiative; for example, the establishment of a task force by the CCME in early 1973 to study the problem and make recommendations to the CCME. Many of the specialty societies were gathering data and analyzing their own specialties; for example, the Study on Surgical Services for the United States (SOSSUS). Those developments prompted the following plea:

The American Board of Medical Specialties believes earnestly that the Federal Government, rather than assuming a primary responsibility for resolving the problems related to health manpower, can best serve the public by supporting the intense and prodigious efforts of the medical profession, medical institutions, and professional organizations responsible for education and health services.[r]

Even acerbic critics of the profession would concede that medical expertise must be a major input into decisions about optimal specialty distribution. Such decisions inherently involve long-range planning; residency quotas set in the middle 1970s will not make an impact on specialty distribution until the 1980s, a fact that requires estimating what health-care demand will be at that time. Health-care demand, however, is to a critical extent the creature of public policy. In some ultimate sense specialty configuration is not exclusively—perhaps not even primarily—a medical issue. There is nothing in a physician's training that makes him peculiarly competent for decision making in that larger sphere; in fact; individual and collective professional interests may bend him, consciously or unconsciously, toward career- or profession-serving rather than toward public-serving postures.

The House committee bill cedes the public's authority to the profession, specifically to professional collectives that contributed heavily to the worsening situation whose amelioration they are asked to devise. To put it differently: In the time-honored American tradition, the regulated and the regulators would be the same persons with different hats.[s] Before passing the committee bill, however, the House deleted the section on specialty distribution, thereby abstaining from the controversy over who should decide the nation's medical

---

[r]Representatives of the five organizations appeared together at the *Hearings*. Their testimony begins at II, 1530. The quote is at 1533.

[s]This perspective was stated to the committee by the HEW secretary in a letter dated March 10, 1975, and included in House Committee Report, p. 76.

specialty mix. The Senate committee quickly reengaged the issue head-on, reporting a bill that provides for "a phase-up to 50 percent of new physicians to enter primary care specialties." If that goal is not met collectively by the medical schools on a voluntary basis, each medical school must meet the goal as a condition for receiving federal capitation grants.

Because AAMC representatives had protested that medical schools often cannot control residency programs, the approach outlined in the bill would deal directly with the sponsoring hospitals in modifying the number and kinds of residencies. A national council and ten regional councils on postgraduate physician training would assist in the planning. The national council would make a thorough study of the whole specialty-training complex, assess needs and the resources required to meet them, and then, after two years, begin to determine on an annual basis the number of residencies to be certified. For the year beginning July 1979, that figure is not to exceed 140 percent of the medical degrees granted in the preceding 12 months.

Social Control of the Specialty Mix

Of particular interest here is the membership of the national and regional councils. Four seats on the national council are to be assigned by the director of the NIH, the medical director of the VA, the assistant secretary for health and environment of the Department of Defense, and an individual chosen by the HEW Secretary. These four persons will name their representatives on the regional councils. The other 20 seats in each case are to be distributed as follows: 12 MDs, 4 nonphysician health professionals, 1 medical student, and 3 representatives of the general public. Of the 12 MDs, 6 are to be practicing physicians, 2 associated with other training centers, and 2 actively engaged in postgraduate training. The 4 nonphysician professionals are to be 2 administrators from hospitals with training programs, 1 health planner or public health administrator, and 1 nurse or allied health practitioner.

Although the five professional organizations that created the LCGME and the CCME are to be consulted by the HEW Secretary about nominations to the councils, those organizations are not to make the decisions about specialty numbers and mix. Moreover, although physicians are to comprise the councils' majorities, the MD component is diverse; and there is substantial representation of the federal bureaucracy and the general public. A primary function of the regional councils is the intraregional allocation of residency positions once the national council has determined the interregional distribution. Clearly the Senate bill politicizes rather than professionalizes the determination of the country's specialty mix. The councils would be federal entities, and the staff would be federal employees.

It is not surprising that the proposal has encountered a great deal of professional antipathy, as well as strong opposition from the Ford administration and many members of Congress. According to two dissenting members of the committee, Senators Beall and Taft, who wrote a supplement to the committee report, the committee proposal is certain to be struck down by the full Senate again, as it was in 1974.

In focusing on the means of regulating physician supply, this discussion has ignored many factors, such as the way in which medical care delivery and payment are organized, which help to determine the number of physicians needed. The development of new kinds of health professionals, called "physician extenders" emerged, largely through pioneering efforts at a handful of medical schools, in the middle and late 1960s. Between 1969 and 1975 HEW funded approximately 100 training programs for physician's assistants, medex, primex, nurse-midwives, and pediatric nurse practitioners, at a cost of about $34,000,000.[t] The quantities and kinds of physician extenders to be trained, the content of their training, whether and how they will be used by delivery systems, and other such issues remain predominantly a matter of physician preference, either collectively or individually; moreover, few safeguards have been erected to ensure that cost reductions or other advantages resulting from the use of physician extenders will be shared with consumers of health care in the form of lower prices.[u]

Market Competition and the HMOs

The Health Maintenance Organization and Resources Act of 1973 was a seminal piece of legislation because, for the first time, the federal government attempted directly to influence the structural and institutional organization of health-care delivery in the private sector. The purpose was to make the market more competitive, as a contribution to cost containment.

---

[t]Data supplied to the national advisory committee established in early 1975 to counsel the National Center for Health Services Research (an HEW agency) concerning a study it had been directed to make of physician-extender selection, training, and deployment. The author is a member of that committee.

[u]The 1972 Amendments to the Social Security Act directed HEW to study Medicare reimbursement patterns with a view to developing a satisfactory way of remunerating physicians for services rendered by their physician-extender employees. That study was delayed but is now in progress. The Social Security Administration, which administers Medicare, had become concerned about billings from doctors, at their regular fees, for services not performed by the physician himself. This raises the interesting issue of whether a fee should attach to the service or to the provider. When the SSA in 1971 declined to reimburse physicians for PA services to Medicare patients, a parodoxical situation emerged: One federal agency in effect rejected the potentially cost-reducing or cost-containing contribution of personnel whose training was being encouraged and funded by another federal agency.

The feature that most clearly distinguishes the HMO from the dominant, traditional delivery system is prepayment for comprehensive health care as opposed to purchase of individual medical services for a fee; prepayment usually takes the form of monthly rates set by an annual contract. What distinguishes HMOs from traditional health-insurance organizations such as Blue Cross and Blue Shield, which also entail prepayment, is the fact that HMO members make contracted payments to the health-care organization itself, in advance, rather than having a third party do so retrospectively, on a fee basis. The motivational implications are obvious. Whereas fee-for-service arrangements embody incentives for overutilization, prepayment discourages overtreatment. Whereas third-party payment externalizes costs and militates against fiduciary responsibility, the HMO tends to nurture cost-consciousness.

Although the term health maintenance organization first surfaced in 1970, HMO prototypes—such as Kaiser-Permanente, Group Health Cooperative of the Puget Sound, and Health Insurance Plan (HIP) of New York—originated during World War II or in the early postwar era. They have been concentrated on the East and West coasts, but during the early 1970s HMOs grew in other urban, high-income areas where their growth was not discouraged by state law.[v] The Nixon administration had embraced the HMO concept as a cost-containment instrument, and the HMO also had friends in both houses of Congress.

Marketeers versus Reformers

HMO supporters can be simplistically divided into market enthusiasts and political reformers. The marketeers believe the best way to protect the interests of consumers and taxpayers is to make the health-care market more competitive. To the degree that the traditional fee-for-service system with its overlay of third-party payment is inefficient, competition from cost-conscious HMOs would tend to lower prices paid by consumers for their own care and by taxpayers for medical services to the indigent. The political reformers, on the other hand, are more interested in providing a certain level and quality of health care to the nation's citizens, even if it must be subsidized by public funds—with whatever redistribution of income, through the tax structure, that approach might entail.

In the congressional deliberations the House committee seemed more responsive to the market perspective and the Senate committee to the social-reform

---

[v]Actually, state legal restrictions probably have been overemphasized as a barrier to HMOs prior to 1973, when the federal HMO act neutralized state constraints. See R. McNeil, Jr. and R.E. Schlenker, "HMOs, Competition, and Government," *Milbank Memorial Fund Quarterly*, 53 (Spring, 1975), 198–200.

perspective.[w] The purpose of this discussion is to show how conflict between the market and the reformist-regulatory approaches was resolved ambiguously in the 1973 act, and to point out some of the implications of that ambiguity for price and cost containment.

The HMO act of December 1973 provided certain benefits to and imposed certain requirements on prepaid-health systems that receive federal certification as HMOs. The most important stimulus to HMOs was the stipulation that all employers of 25 or more persons who pay part of their employees' health costs must offer an HMO option if a certified HMO is available. That provision enhanced consumer choice, and the fact that HMOs were permitted to advertise the nonprofessional aspects of their services was a contribution to the market principle of consumer knowledge. In defining a certifiable HMO, however, the act departed sharply from the "fair-market" principle that HMOs should be able to compete without subsidy.

The House committee approach was more permissive in defining a certifiable HMO; that is, less inclined to encumber HMOs with reformist requirements that would make price competition with non-HMOs more difficult. The House bill therefore contained less generous subsidies in the form of grants, loans, and loan guarantees. The Senate bill, in contrast, loaded requirements onto HMOs. Benefits offered by HMOs to their subscribers had to include—in addition to comprehensive preventive and treatment services, inpatient and outpatient—a list of services not typically offered even by existing HMOs, for example, preventive dentistry for children, and aid for alcoholism, drug-abuse, and mental health problems. One-third of the HMO's board of directors must be enrollees (consumer voice), membership in the HMO must be representative of the community, there must be total-family participation, and certain quality-assurance[x] and continuing education programs must be pursued. Perhaps the most challenging requirements were open enrollment and community rating. A certified HMO, for a period of at least 30 days per year, must accept individual applicants, in the order in which they apply, up to the HMO's capacity. No consideration can be given to the health status of the applicants. That requirement, coupled with the stipulation that a general rate (for example, the monthly membership payment) apply to all subscribers—rather than varying rates among subscriber groups according to risk differentials—is particularly hard for an HMO to meet and still keep its prices competitive without subsidy. Indeed, the Senate bill

---

[w]The committees that drafted the HMO legislation were the same as for the medical manpower legislation discussed the section "Medical Subsidies."

[x]There has been some criticism of HMOs as a threat to quality because of the financial incentive to cut utilization rates. However, there is little evidence for that view. See M.I. Roemer and W. Shonick, "HMO Performance: the Recent Evidence," *Milbank Memorial Fund* Quarterly, 51 (Summer, 1973), 271–317.

included subsidies estimated at over $5 billion; moreover, proponents of the Senate committee approach pointed to what was then perceived as the imminence of national health insurance, which could have been the source of other funding for HMOs.

The compromise eventually reached cut the Senate figures for program subsidies drastically and provided only modest planning, evaluation, and administrative funds—$375 million over five years. Yet the act left the benefit package and other requirements essentially intact, and the first cost estimates of those requirements suggested to many observers that the certifiable HMO might have been priced out of the market. After all, many of the expensive requirements placed upon HMOs were not required of fee-for-service systems or health-insurance agencies.

The act pleased neither reformers nor marketeers. An especially forceful critique of the HMO act from the marketeering perspective was given by Professor Clark C. Havighurst in his testimony at the Senate Judiciary Committee's antitrust hearings on the health-care system in the spring of 1974. Here are some of his comments:

. . . a handful of people on Capitol Hill saw this as an opportunity to write their ideal of a health care system into law. Their idea was to "restructure the system," as the current phrase goes, to organize the delivery of care to a degree never attempted in the past. . . . Fearing that the HMO of their dreams would never happen if one counted on private initiatives and investments to produce it, they have dedicated a substantial amount of federal money to subsidize its realization. . . . If their idea is a good one, why wouldn't it happen without subsidies? If the answer is that the health care marketplace is a faulty one, why not correct its faults so that their idea can have a fair test against the competition?

I hope it is clear that I am not being critical of the HMO idea per se. Indeed, I consider myself one of its most enthusiastic champions. . . . The essence of an HMO is not the comprehensiveness of the benefits it offers, its particular mode of organization, or its grandiosity in size. It is provider prepayment alone that sets it apart. This financing system changes incentives of providers in important ways, and this change in incentives is alone sufficient to account for the success which some HMOs have experienced over a long period of time.[y]

The first HMO certification came in the fall of 1975, and by the late spring of 1976 about a dozen had occurred. Meanwhile there was considerable pressure from HMOs and their supporters to amend the original act to permit HMOs to become more competitive without heavy subsidy. At this writing, House and Senate conferees are reviewing the proposals of respective bills that would

---

[y]*Competition In The Health Services Market*, Hearings before the Subcommittee on Antitrust and Monopoly, Senate Committee on the Judiciary, 93rd Congress, 2nd Session, May, 1974, Part 2, 1078. Professor Havighurst's presentation begins at 1036 and includes two published papers on the health-care market.

soften somewhat the original act's provisions concerning the benefit package, open enrollment, community rating, and several other requirements. To the degree that HMOs can be made more independently competitive, the market as a decision maker will be strengthened.[z]

HMOs and Medicare

The 1973 act prohibited an HMO from raising its enrollment of indigents, including Medicare and Medicaid participants, to more than 75 percent of its membership, but in granting assistance to new HMOs the government had to give preference to HMOs that accept such groups for enrollment. One would suppose that, given the enthusiasm for the cost-efficiency of HMOs expressed by the White House as early as 1970, strong efforts would have been made to get Medicaid and Medicare beneficiaries enrolled in existing HMOs even before the HMO act of 1975. On the contrary, efforts in that direction appear to have been casual in spite of some encouragement from the Congress in the 1972 Social Security Act amendments, which permitted states to use HMOs for Medicaid recipients. Medicare, more directly under federal administration, has failed to take advantage of the HMO's prepayment incentives to provide care more efficiently by reducing unnecessary use. Essentially, the federal government has bought services from HMOs, for the small number of Medicare participants who have enrolled in HMOs, on a cost-reimbursement rather than a membership-rate basis, as though the HMO were a fee-for-service system.

This policy provides yet another example of the ambiguity of federal initiatives in addressing the question of whether primary reliance should be placed in market, profession, or federal regulators for a particular kind of decision. On the one hand the Congress encourages HMOs—and the market as a decision maker—by requiring employers to offer an HMO alternative to employees; on the other hand the federal bureaucracy, in buying care for the elderly and the poor with tax dollars, declines to take advantage of the very cost-efficiency possibilities that caused Congress to encourage HMOs in the first place.

Conclusion

The purpose in discussing PSROs, subsidies for medical education, and HMOs was to illustrate persistent ambiguities in the allocation of decision making

---

[z]For a thorough exposition of the issue of HMO competitiveness, see the paper issued by the Institute of Medicine, National Academy of Sciences, "HMOs: Toward a Fair Market Test," Washington, D.C., 1974.

At this writing, more than a dozen HMOs have been certified, and amendments to the HMO Act which would make some of the original requirements (e.g., in re open enrollment) less burdensome appear to be near passage.

among market, profession, and federal bureau, and to point out some of the price and cost implications of those ambiguities. Equivocation about the location of authority is only one of the many drags upon cost-efficiency; the roots of price inflation in the medical industry are complex and the solutions elusive. Cost containment would be a challenge even if the loci of decision were clearly and optimally arranged. Yet it seems certain that clouded and inconsistent lines of authority not only exacerbate inflationary pressures but encumber remedial action.

The price and cost consequences were more predictable for some of the earlier federal initiatives than for more recent programs. It was fairly obvious, for instance, that, given the inability of physician supply to respond quickly, Medicare-Medicaid's sudden stimulus to demand would bring price inflation unless effective price monitoring were established. The net price and cost consequences of the PSROs, in contrast, are more difficult to forecast, because the PSRO initiative contains countervailing price and cost thrusts. Even so, there are moral as well as cost-rationalization purposes to be served by a cleaner engagement of the authority-allocation issue. Many of the most challenging questions that confront medical-care policy makers in the 1970s would be unanswerable by objective criteria, even if all of the data were in—because they are at root questions of value judgment or preference.

Only an overarching approach to the whole range of medical-care issues would permit a satisfactory determination of the kinds of decisions best made, *from the public interest perspective*, by profession or market as opposed to government bureau. Only such an overview, plus a commitment to consistency, would prevent ambiguities, nonsequiturs, and discrepancies, within and among federal programs, such as those exemplified by the failure of Medicare administrators to use the advantages of HMOs, or by continued purchase of hospital services on an essentially cost-plus basis instead of by contractual prices set in advance. In both of these examples a federal establishment that characterizes itself as committed in general to exploiting the competitive market as an instrument of price- and cost-containment is engaging in behavior that ignores, even flouts, a cardinal principle of the market, namely, reliance on private initiative's enlightened self-interest to reduce costs below the contractual price.

Such inconsistencies are not, of course, attributable solely to oversight, short-sightedness, or a failure of reason. Ambiguities often serve political needs. One way for Congress to handle the cross-pressures of conflicting interest groups is to give something to everyone, or to camouflage lines of authority; or even to create intentionally an ambiguous situation in which the ultimate victor is unpredictable at the time of the legislative action, in which case each interest group may be willing to "go along" because it has a fighting chance to come out ahead. Given the political context in which the question of decision locus must be engaged, it is not surprising that ambiguities and inconsistencies burden attempts to deal with price inflation.

One general development seems solidly based, however. The relative insensitivity to costs that characterized so much of the legislation in this field 10 or 15 years ago—when the overwhelming challenge was to marshall enough resources to meet the jump in demand—is no more. Congress and the White House have been forced into acute cost-consciousness by inflation in the medical sphere. In meeting this new challenge the government and the polity have moved far beyond the old assumption that incentives internal to market and profession will bring their behavior into consonance with the common good. In the new national mood, which requires public accountability of the medical profession and competitiveness of the market, particularly when public monies are expended, the day of the federal regulator seems to have arrived.

The Limits of Regulation: Implications of Alternative Models for the Health Sector

Bruce C. Vladeck

The debate over government regulation of the health sector illustrates the limitations of incremental policy making. Alarmed by the seemingly uncontrollable drain on public funds created by health-care costs, Congress and the executive branch grope for whatever straws seem available. Leaders of the hospital industry and—to a lesser extent—of organized medicine try to forestall a loss of their autonomous power by creating or reinforcing government-sanctioned cartelization. Academics and policy analysts make a virtue of the inadequacy of positive policy theory by shooting the proposals of both groups full of holes, offering as an alternative only the purely imaginary characteristics of an idealized free market. The three groups increasingly talk past one another, able to agree only on the proposition that the existing state of affairs is untenable, and that no one can agree on the best way to get out of it.

Without pretending to have identified the one best way, this chapter attempts a more "synoptic" approach to the problem. By scanning a somewhat broader and more generalized range of techniques for achieving the goals of public policy, it seeks to refocus the discussion of health-sector regulation. Instead of making a fragmented series of "limited successive comparisons," it begins by posing this question: Given the seemingly available alternatives, what is the best we can do, and is it any better than what we now have?

In this sense, what follows constitutes an effort to take seriously Randall Ripley's contention that public policy analysis comprises the study of alternative techniques of government action.[1] If policy analysis has anything to offer to policy choice, it is the recognition that defining desired outcomes is not enough to produce them. Different means of "production" lead to different outcomes. Although the study of public policy is not now—and may never be—sophisticated enough to provide determinate solutions to the problem of choosing among techniques, it may still contribute something just by defining the problem as one of that kind of choice. By proceeding in this way I hope, therefore, not only to cast some feeble light on the particular policy issue at hand—regulation of the health sector—but also to demonstrate the potential utility of a *political* science of policy analysis.

Four agglomerations of techniques—called models, although classes or ideal-types might have been just as accurate a term—are described and compared. They are utility regulation, licensing, law enforcement, and contracting. Like all names, these are somewhat arbitrary, but the choice of these models is not. Not only do they encompass a substantial part of the spectrum of regulatory tools with which there is extensive experience in the United States, but they are different enough from one another to make comparisons useful. Through those comparisons, and a comparison of all four alternatives with existing reality, it is possible to suggest some conclusions about most- and least-desirable techniques of regulation for health sector.

Regulation: A Definition

In Theodore Lowi's famous typology of policy processes, regulative policies are those that apply the threat of coercion to individual conduct, rather than to the environment of conduct, and in which the likelihood of coercion is immediate rather than remote.[2]   In other words, regulative policies apply or threaten to apply sanctions, rather than rewards, to identifiable individuals and groups, rather than to more generalized classes or components of the population. There are serious shortcomings to Lowi's definition. For one, it defies operational-ization.[3] More to the point, many policies adopted by agencies generally thought of as regulatory fall into Lowi's three other categories. Nonetheless, Lowi's definition of regulation is adopted here, primarily for the virtues of what it excludes. Although tax incentives and disincentives, subsidies with no real strings attached, and hortatory statements by public officials are all in some sense regulatory, in that they constitute attempts by public officials to alter the behavior of private firms and individuals, they are not considered. Most of the debate and policy experimentation on regulation in the health field has been concentrated on actions falling into Lowi's regulative category. Although the range of theoretically possible policy choices is infinite, the effective range of choice tends to be far more circumscribed, and in this instance a relatively narrow construction or regulation is appropriate.

The Crisis in Health Care

The thrust towards greater government regulation of health services arises primarily from a single source: astronomical increases in cost. Total expenditures for health services have more than tripled since 1965, exceeding $118 billion in fiscal year 1975. Over the last ten years, the average annual rate of increase has exceeded 10 percent, and the proportion of the Gross National Product devoted to health care has grown from 5.9 to 8.3 percent. More directly tied to the thrust towards regulation is the disproportionate part of those increases that has been drawn from public funds. Since the introduction of Medicare and Medicaid, the governmental share of expenditures for *personal* health care has increased from 21 to almost 40 percent, and in absolute amounts has gone from just under $7 billion to over $40 billion. Most of that increase has come from federal funds.[a]

Because they involve "entitlement" programs and because, with the possible exception of Medicaid, those programs are politically popular, the annually mandated increases in government health spending constitute a major "uncontrollable" constraint on the budget. As such, they are a source of considerable distress and concern, and methods for controlling the uncontrollable have been increasingly sought.[b]

Private citizens, of course, have hardly been unaffected by the spiral of medical costs, and their elected representatives are undoubtedly sensitive to their concerns. But the demand for regulation in the health sector differs from that which characterized the imposition of utility-style regulation on other sectors of the economy. There, high prices combined with public hostility towards the profits of "monopolists" generated the demand for regulation.[c] In the health sector, on the other hand, the desire for regulation—apart from the hospital industry's own interest—appears to originate largely in governmental rather than popular attitudes; policy initiative, in other words, is flowing downwards, rather than upwards. Moreover, "monopoly profits" can hardly be said to characterize the nonprofit hospital industry—the subtleties of surpluses or wasteful expenditures as surrogate forms of monopoly return to institutions probably escape most citizens and many of their representatives—and public hostility to rising physician fees and incomes has not generated much in the way of political pressure.

Instead, popular demands on the political system relative to health care largely continue to take the form of a desire for more and better care. Legislators are sympathetic, but budget constraints — reinforced by the new congressional budgeting procedure — make new initiatives impossible until costs are brought under control. Thus Congress has become preoccupied with regulation, not from a desire to indulge punitive attitudes towards health-care providers, but from a recognition that, without regulation-induced change, Americans will not be able to afford the health services they want.[4]

---

[a]All these figures are derived from Marjorie Smith Mueller and Robert M. Gibson, "National Health Expenditures, Fiscal Year 1975," 39, *Social Security Bulletin* (February 1976), pp. 3–20, 48.

[b]On "uncontrollability," see Barry M. Blechman, Edward M. Gramlich, and Robert W. Hartman, *Setting National Priorities: The 1975 Budget* (Washington: The Brookings Institution), 1974, pp. 26–29.

[c]Or reinforced that created by the affected firms themselves. Cf. Marver H. Bernstein, *Regulating Business by Independent Commission* (Princeton, N.J.: Princeton University Press), 1955, pp. 21ff.; Richard A. Posner, "Natural Monopoly and its Regulation," 21, *Stanford Law Review* (February, 1969), pp. 620–622; but compare Gabriel Kolko, *Railroads and Regulation, 1877-1916* (Princeton: Princeton University Press), 1965.

Structural Characteristics of the Health Industry

Just what has caused the rapid increases in health costs and expenditures is a complex and controversial subject, largely outside the scope of this chapter. There are, however, seven structural characteristics of the health industry that are, by general agreement, felt to be tied to the cost problem, and that are also central to any consideration of alternative regulatory techniques. The relative contribution of each of these characteristics to the cost-price problem is not, in other words, at issue here, but it is necessary at least to describe them in order to talk sensibly about regulatory alternatives.

The Nature of Demand. First, of course, is the unique nature of the demand for health services. Only 33 percent of all expenditures for personal-health services represent direct out-of-pocket payments by consumers; for hospital care, where "unit cost" is the highest and where the largest single chunk of total health expenditures is consumed, only 8 percent of all expenses are met out of pocket by consumers.[5] The low incremental cost of many services to consumers thus creates an extremely low price elasticity of demand for many services.

Moreover, an extremely large proportion of demand is provider, rather than consumer generated. Physicians determine who will be admitted to hospitals, how long patients will stay, when they will be discharged, and what services they will receive when there. They make all the decisions about the use of prescription drugs, which comprise 10 percent of total national health-care costs. They also exercise considerable control over the frequency of ambulatory services, especially for patients with chronic illnesses.[d] Increased consumer skepticism towards physicians notwithstanding, this pervasive control of demand by suppliers is more often sought than resisted. When ill, most of us are just as happy to transfer the burdens of decision making to the occupant of the still quasi-mystical role of physician.

Oligopsony. The principal counterbalance to physician-managed demand has thus increasingly become, in recent years, not individual consumers but the third parties that now pick up most of the costs (even though those costs are eventually passed on to consumers). Indeed, another crucial characteristic of the health-care industry for purposes of evaluating regulatory devices is the increasing movement towards monopsony—or at least oligopsony. That means that certain components of the health-care market are increasingly dominated by a single or several buyers. For hospital services, the monopsonist is generally Blue Cross,

---

[d]Victor Fuchs, especially, emphasizes the role of physicians in health-care costs. See Victor R. Fuchs, *Who Shall Live?: Health, Economics, and Social Choice* (New York: Basic Books), 1974, pp. 59-61.

as an agent both for its own subscribers and, through the role of fiscal intermediary, federally insured individuals. In many poor urban communities, the government itself is increasingly a monopsonist. Should national health insurance ever arrive, the government may, of course, have nearly complete monopsony power, either directly or through private agents.

"Natural Monopoly." In many parts of the country, these monopsonists will confront "natural monopolies." Although there are over 6,000 short-term community hospitals in the United States, the market for health-care services is highly localized. Given the economies of scale in hospital operations, there are many markets in which the economically efficient number of facilities would be, at most, a handful. Although physicians are more numerous in most communities, the cartelization created by licensure and professional societies often permits them to behave as monopolists as well.[6]

Other characteristics of natural monopoly also pervade the health sector. For hospital-based services, and to a lesser but not insignificant extent physician services, economies of scale create falling marginal-cost curves all the way out to the limit of optimal efficient capacity. Total costs of operating a hospital with a 90 percent occupancy rate, in other words, are not significantly greater than those of running the same hospital at 60 percent occupancy.[7]

Labor Intensiveness. Paradoxically, declining marginal cost in the health industry is not a result, as in other natural monopolies, of capital intensiveness. Indeed, health care, like most services, is highly labor intensive.[8] Although the total social investment in physical plant in the health sector is enormous, and a major source of concern for those seeking to develop new regulator devices, the cost implications of new investment lie more in the labor costs inevitably associated with them than in the costs of the facilities themselves. Unlike manufacturing or utility industries, capital investment in health tends to increase the demand for labor, rather than to substitute for it.[9]

Rapid Technological Change. That phenomenon, in turn arises at least partially from the extremely rapid rate of technological change in the health industry. Public investment in biomedical research and development is exceeded only by that in the defense sector, and the diffusion of innovations in health care—encouraged by the absence of constraints on the demand side—has been especially rapid.[10] The effective life cycle for new plant and equipment is thus much shorter than in industries like surface transportation or electric power.

Unavailability of Substitutes. In theory, those natural monopolies generally described as public utilities are characterized by what economists might call the unavailability of substitutes. Substitution is potentially an important check on monopoly power; if the oil trust exacts monopoly prices, consumers may be induced to switch to coal or firewood for heating their homes, and the very threat of that substitution should keep the oil trust in line. Critics of public regulation have recently come to question the extent to which satisfactory substitutes really are available in many of those industries long thought to be natural monopolies, although their arguments are not entirely convincing.[11] But it is certainly true that most consumers feel there are no satisfactory substitutes for certain aspects of medical care. Although at the margins high prices may induce some consumers to adopt substitutes like self-care, those with potentially disabling or fatal conditions susceptible to pharmacological or surgical intervention are unlikely to find alternatives within the marketplace. Much has been made in recent years of substitution *within* the health sector— of outpatient for inpatient care, of visits to physicians' assistants rather than physicians—and these are important trends; but in many instances there truly is no substitute for a highly trained physician working within a well-equipped hospital.

Ubiquity of Market Discrimination. Physicians have customarily used sliding fee scales in which their more prosperous (or least-favored) patients subsidized the poorer (or more favored) ones. Although reimbursement mechanisms under government third-party payment programs have provided a powerful disincentive for those sliding scales, price discrimination continues, often in other forms. The even more massive cross-subsidization practiced by hospitals has been sanctioned, at least indirectly, by third-party payers. Surgical patients continue to subsidize obstetrical ones; pharmacies subsidize nurseries; and well-insured patients undergoing routine elective procedures subsidize indigent emergency cases.[e]

Moreover, both physicians and hospitals continue to retain considerable discretion over whom they will provide services to. Even a citizen of a metropolitan area with an overabundance of facilities will generally lack a free choice of hospitals to select from, being limited instead to those that provide admitting privileges to his physician. In a far different situation, the implementation of Medicaid in many areas has been hampered by the unwillingness of physicians to treat Medicaid patients. Teaching hospitals, although to a far lesser extent than formerly, continue to admit service patients on the basis of the interestingness of their conditions, rather than on purely "market" considerations; beds sit empty on specialty wards while nearby public hospitals are overcrowded.

---

[e]The most lucid discussion of cross-subsidization in hospital charges I have encountered can be found in Sylvia Law, *Blue Cross: What Went Wrong?* (New Haven: Yale University Press), 1974, pp. 74–89. Cf. also Roger G. Noll, "The Consequences of Public Utility Regulation of Hospitals," in Institute of Medicine, National Academy of Sciences, *Controls on Health Care,* Proceedings of the Conference on Regulation in the Health Industry, January 7-9, 1974 (Washington: National Academy of Sciences), 1975, pp. 40–41; and Clark C. Havighurst, "Regulation of Health Facilities and Services by 'Certificate of Need'," 59, *Virginia Law Review* (October 1973), p. 1191.

Dominance of Nonprofit Institutions. No one knows quite what to make of the predominance of voluntary, not-for-profit institutions. The small body of theory on the economic behavior of such institutions suggests that their pricing behavior may not be radically different from that which profit-maximizing firms may adopt, but not-for-profits obviously do not distribute returns on capital to shareholders. What they do with surpluses is an interesting question—and an important one for regulatory design; one especially convincing hypothesis is that much of it flows to prestige-generating, surplus-consuming putative quality improvements.[12] When combined with the continued preponderance of solo practice or partnership arrangements for physicians, however, the not-for-profit status of most hospitals means that throughout the health sector—with the significant but hardly central exceptions of pharmaceutical and equipment manufacturers, proprietary hospitals and nursing homes, and private insurance companies—the enormous volume of health expenditures creates relatively little return to capital. Most goes, instead, to labor, especially the uniquely high-priced labor of physicians. At the very least, the health sector as a whole is, therefore, a particularly inappropriate site for price regulation based on "reasonable rate of return" to invested capital.[f]

Structural Characteristics: Summary. In summary, then, the principal economic characteristics of the health industry of relevance to regulatory policy are these:

1. The low price elasticity of demand for many kinds of services, resulting in part from the high proportion of third-party payments, the extent to which demand is controlled by sellers, and the unavailability of adequate substitutes for many kinds of services
2. The strong trend towards monopsony, or at least oligopsony, in the market for major kinds of services
3. Increasing returns to scale in an industry of highly localized markets, leading, in some communities, to natural monopolies or oligopolies in the supply of hospital services, and to declining marginal costs in a broader range of services
4. Labor intensiveness
5. Rapid technological change
6. Unavailability of substitutes
7. Pervasive price and other forms of market discrimination with extensive concomitant cross-subsidization
8. The extremely limited role of returns to capital, related to the still somewhat mysterious behavior of not-for-profit voluntary institutions

---

[f]The nursing-home subsector may constitute an exception. Cf. Bruce C. Vladeck, "Public Utility Regulation and the Nursing Homes: We Know the Answer, What's the Question?" *Proceedings,* National Conference on Long-Term Care Reimbursement (Silver Spring, Md.: Applied Management Sciences, Inc.), forthcoming.

Each of these characteristics must be adequately considered and accounted for in the evaluation of alternative regulatory techniques.

Four Models of Regulation

Although much of the contemporary debate about regulation in the health sector revolves around what is described here as the utility regulation model, the conglomeration of activities that comprise utility regulation constitute only a small part of the total spectrum of available regulatory techniques. As Anne Somers has so eloquently pointed out, the arsenal of government regulation contains an almost infinite supply of infinitely varied alternatives.[g]

Confronted by complexity, the instinctive response of a researcher is to fall back on that process of abstraction described as "modelling," to create some order in the subject matter, no matter how limited or arbitrary. The four models discussed here are subject to all the limitations inherent in that abstracting process. The extent to which any actual government agency conforms in any detail with any of these models is somewhat problematic. For utility regulation alone, the range of actual variation includes at least 7 federal agencies and 51 (including the District of Columbia) state agencies that often resemble one another only in name. The ingenuity of legislators is formidable, as is their willingness to combine administrative functions and statutory responsibilities willy-nilly in individual agencies. But to do comparative analysis one must have *something* to compare. The four models presented here were therefore constructed with a dual purpose. On the other hand, it was more important that they each be internally consistent, and that they differ from one another in as many important descriptive characteristics as possible. (See summary, table 6-1.)

Model I: Utility Regulation

The first and most familiar model is called utility "regulation." Its primary characteristics are as follows:[h]

---

[g]Well-summarized in Anne R. Somers, "Regulation of Hospitals," 400, *The Annals* (March 1972), pp. 69-81.

[h]This model has been drawn primarily from James W. McKie, "The Ends and Means of Regulation," General Series Reprint 287 (Washington: The Brookings Institution), 1974; Bernstein, *Regulating Business by Independent Commission;* William M. Capron, "Introduction," to Capron, ed., *Technological Change in Regulated Industries,* Studies in the Regulation of Economic Activity (Washington: The Brookings Institution), 1971, pp. 2-3; A.J.G. Priest, "Possible Adaptation of Public Utility Concepts in the Health Care Field," 35, *Law and Contemporary Problems* (Autumn 1970), pp. 839-848; and American Hospital Association, "Report of the Advisory Panel on Public Utility Regulation," April 27, 1971; but is in total agreement, of course, with none of them.

Table 6-1
Summary of Characteristics of Regulatory Models

Model	(a) Administrative Structure	(b) Primary Focus	(c) Secondary Focus	(d) Impact on Entry	(e) Characteristics of Process	(f) Enforcement
I. *Utility Regulation* Examples: ICC, CAB, FCC, FPC, and state agency counterparts	Specialized agency, often multiheaded; operating under broad but vague mandate	Rates (behavior) mandatory jurisdiction, but otherwise high discretion.	Other aspects of behavior; substantial discretion	Discouraging	Low visibility in spite of trappings of due process and public notice	An afterthought despite broad discretion
II. *Licensing* Examples: State Departments of health; New York State Board of Regents; Certificate of need agencies	Specialized agency, generally with interest-group representation or domination at the state level	Qualifications (inputs) through highly nondiscretionary administration of "objective" criteria	"Moral character and fitness"	Highly discouraging in practice; potential for encouraging entry exists	Low visibility except in scandals	Reliance on self-policing by professionals; revocation an awkward tool
III. *Law Enforcement* Examples: FDA, OSHA, Wage and Hours Division (Dept. of Labor)	Bureaucratic hierarchy, heavily reliant on specific standards and information gathering	Detailed specification of conduct (behavior), often with considerable technical complexity; maximal discretion	Narrow focus limits secondary impact	Little impact	Intermittent visibility; substantial publicity alternates with apparent disappearance	Severe difficulties in optimizing resource allocation to enforcement
IV. *Contracting* Examples: NIH, OE, Department of Defense procurement; Energy Research & Development Administration & predecessor components of AEC	Regulatory activities secondary to primary bureaucratic activity	Detailed specification of items (output); enormous discretion notwithstanding bureaucratic constraints	The core of contracting as a regulatory activity; wide range of focuses and enormous discretion	Can either encourage or discourage	Low visibility except in scandals	Enforcement through termination largely self-defeating; heavy reliance on bargaining results

1. It is administered by a body charged solely with the regulation of a certain industry, or set of industries, often but not invariably a multiheaded, collegial group of commissioners or administrators, operating under a broad legislative grant of administrative discretion providing no more than general guidelines for the regulators.

2. Its primary focus is the prices or rates charged by firms in the regulated industry or industries. Whether or not prior approval by the regulator is required, it retains power over all rates and charges, subject to the constraints of statutory and constitutional law—the latter mandating, in the case of private firms, a "reasonable" rate of return on invested capital. Oversight of prices is thus "mandatory" rather than "discretionary," in the sense that the regulatory authority is required by law to do *something* about rates, if only to supervise their filing, although its discretion as to what it does about them may be enormous.

3. Because control of rates alone may produce distortions counterproductive to the other ends for which regulation is generally sought, regulatory authorities tend to mandate requirements related to other aspects of the firm's behavior. Most common are standards of service or quality, although accounting techniques, capital financing and expenditure decisions, and purchasing policies are often included. In this and other respects, utility regulation is inherently expansionary, at least partially as a result of what James McKie has called the "tar-baby" effect; regulation of one aspect of a firm's behavior tends to create distortions in other aspects, thus generating the impetus for still more regulation in a self-reinforcing cycle.[13]

4. Because rate regulation in the private sector tends to guarantee a rate of return at least approaching the current cost of capital, and because regulated firms are often required to maintain higher standards of service, or serve less profitable customers, or engage in other sorts of behavior that firms in a purely competitive industry would not, rate regulation must invariably be accompanied by control of entry to the industry. Conversely, the granting of a license of "public convenience and necessity" creates at least potential monopoly power for the grantee, thus implying a need for rate regulation. Customarily, utility regulation extends not only to entry per se, but also to the establishment, maintenance, and discontinuance of service of certain kinds or in certain locales. In many instances, it also extends to mergers and acquisitions.

5. In spite of the obscurity in which it commonly occurs, rate regulation is endowed with the trappings that are supposed to create "visibility" in government action. These include public hearings, frequent use of adversary proceedings, and the creation of an elaborate public record.

6. Determinations of the regulatory authority are presumed to be self-enforcing. Although administrative and statutory provisions for enforcement are often available, the extremely broad range of sanctions available to the regulators and the pervasiveness of their oversight of the regulatees are generally thought to obviate the need for extensive enforcement mechanisms.[14]

Model II: Licensing

Although utility regulation implies control over entry, such controls can be exercised in the absence of the other characteristics of utility regulation. Phrased differently, utility regulation implies licensing, but licensing need not imply utility regulation. Of the four models presented here, licensing is the one with which there has been the most health-sector experience, but its application is hardly limited to health alone. Indeed, licensing, in the form of the granting of exclusive franchises, is perhaps the oldest form of regulation practiced by modern nation-states, preexisting the development of capitalism. In contrast to utility regulation, licensing has tended to focus on quality and standards of services, and has generally demonstrated the following characteristics:[i]

1. Again, licensing is usually administered by an administrative organization specialized either in licensing itself or in a specific industry. In many instances, the licensing authority is identical to the dominant professional association or organization in the industry, as in "unified bar" states or those that vest medical licensure in the state medical association. When the two are not identical, representation of professional groups in the licensing authority is generally mandated.[j] In the United States to date, licensing, as opposed to licensure under federal utility regulation, has been exclusively a state function.

2. The primary focus of licensing is the standards and qualifications of individual entrants to an industry or profession. Standards are maintained through the use of "objective" administrative criteria such as examinations or, more recently, criteria of "need." As a result, licensing, at least in theory, tends to be highly nondiscretionary, as judicial interests in due process have demanded that all those meeting some objective criterion be permitted to apply for licenses, and all who meet further criteria be granted them.

3. Although the rationale of licensing implies an extensive state interest in many characteristics of the behavior of licensees, control of that behavior tends to rely on adherence to the ethical standards of the profession or industry involved, and on licensees' "character and fitness."

---

[i]The licensing model has been drawn primarily from Harris S. Cohen, "Professional Licensure, Organizational Behavior, and the Public Interest," 51, *The Milbank Memorial Fund Quarterly: Health and Society* (Winter, 1973), pp. 73-88; National Advisory Committee on Health Manpower, *Report* (Washington: U.S. Government Printing Office), 1967, Vol. II, Appendix VII; and Herbert L. Packer, *The Limits of the Criminal Sanction* (Stanford, Calif.: Stanford University Press), 1968, pp. 253-256.

[j]Exceptions to this general pattern tend to fall into two categories: for those professions in which completion of defined educational requirements are the primary precondition for licensure, the primary authority may reside in the agency with purview of the state's educational activities, such as the New York State Board of Regents, which supervises licensure for physicians and other medical personnel. In radically different kinds of industries, such as the sale of alcoholic beverages, licensing authorities are often keystones of the state government's patronage structure.

4. Licensing constitutes an absolute control over entry, and is often manipulated in order to maintain the monopoly power of those already possessing licenses, as in the reluctance of most states to honor medical licenses from other states. When the potential supply of high-quality professionals or services is greater than the present supply of licensed providers, however, licensing contains at least the potential of increasing competition by increasing the supply of licenses.

5. Licensing tends to be a relatively nonpublic process, consisting primarily of the relationships between a number of atomistic individuals or small firms and a single administrative body. It is thus characterized by the kind of privatization that typifies relationships between interest groups and government agencies that exist primarily to confer benefits on them.[15] From time to time, however, scandals or other forms of media exposure will force a reinstitution of arm's-length relationships between regulators and regulatees, at least for a while.

6. Under licensing, enforcement is distinctly Janus-faced. On the one hand, severe sanctions, generally including criminal penalties, are provided against those who would compete in licensed industries without licenses, although the vigor with which those sanctions are enforced varies according to the kind of industry involved (in health it tends to be rather stringent) and the jurisdiction. Such enforcement rests with criminal authorities, not the licensing agency itself. Once licensed, however, the individual possessor is largely immune from sanctions. Service standards, ethical behavior, and other characteristics tend to be overseen only through limited, often largely toothless, professional or industry self-regulation. Licenses tend to be either automatically renewable or granted for an indefinite period, and even those requirements written into the license itself are rarely enforced through revocation.

Model III: Law Enforcement

Of the four models, law enforcement has been the most difficult to define, in spite of a strong intuitive feeling that there do indeed exist a coherent body of regulatory activities for which it is appropriate. Those difficulties arose, in retrospect, from two conceptual problems, which should be cleared away here first, lest they cause the reader the same qualms that I was finally able to overcome. First, legal theorists are generally hostile to any confusion between the criminal and civil laws, or between criminal and civil penalties or criminal and civil enforcement mechanisms.[16] Nonetheless, the two processes have enough in common to permit lumping them together. Second, the other models—as indeed most government behavior—also contain provisions for the enforcement of administrative determinations through legal and judicial processes. In this not unreasonable sense, the law-enforcement model might be defined as that regulatory behavior which lacks the special characteristics of the other models, and which consists of the simplest dyad of (1) the formulation of rules and (2) the imposition of sanctions on those who violate them. Yet even that simple process generally implies, in the United States, the following characteristics as well:

1. The classical bifurcation of rule making and ajudication *omits entirely* the central administrative process in law enforcement, which can best be described as "prosecutorial." Prosecutorial agencies are almost necessarily hierarchial bureaucracies, and are necessarily separate from adjudicatory bodies, which in law enforcement tend to be the courts. (This characteristic is important in differentiating law enforcement from utility regulation.) The primary activities of prosecutorial agencies are information gathering and the preparation and presentation of charges, whether in the form of criminal indictments, civil complaints, cease and desist orders, or whatever.

2. Constitutional prohibitions on vagueness, and the technical complexity on the issues with which law-enforcement agencies outside the criminal justice sector must often work, create a reliance on highly detailed and precise standards of conduct—if not in the statute or regulation under which action is brought, at least in the content of the specific action itself. Law-enforcement agencies, by the definitions employed here, are thus confined largely to the enforcement of relatively specific and detailed behavioral rules composed almost exclusively of prohibitions. Regulation through law enforcement is, nonetheless, the most highly discretionary kind of regulation. The prosecutorial function in the criminal justice system, it is increasingly recognized, permits almost total freedom of choice as to who will be regulated and what regulations will be enforced;[17] that freedom of administrative choice is, if anything, even greater in the regulation of industrial or professional conduct in the health sector.

3. Because it revolves largely around the enforcement of prohibitions, the ability of law-enforcement activities to compel affirmative behavior of any kind is extremely limited. Similarly, the narrowness of its focus permits those not anxious to comply to seek to get around regulation through law enforcement by avoiding prohibited behavior to the minimal extent necessary to avoid sanctions. As a result, the standards employed by law-enforcement agencies tend to become "minimum acceptable levels," in Alvin Gouldner's phrase,[18] and a cycle of what might be called "law-enforcement regulatory lag" arises, in which each new form of evasion generates a new set of regulations, with the regulatory agencies perpetually one step behind the regulatees.

4. Because they are so strictly limited to behavior, law-enforcement activities have little impact on regulated firms or individuals apart from the specific conduct specified, and thus have almost no impact on entry or disentry. Whereas violation of a basic condition of licensure may lead to revocation of the license, the finding that a firm has violated the regulations of the Food and Drug Administration or the State Department of Health will rarely have consequences for the firm outside the specific penalties attached to the offending behavior.

5. The relationship of law-enforcement activities to public visibility is bifurcated. On the one hand, information-gathering activities are highly dependent on secrecy, as a means both of securing cooperation and or maximizing the impact of deterrence. Dramatic public exposure, on the other hand, is not only the most effective sanction the law-enforcement agency can bring to bear itself, but is also crucial to institutional maintenance and survival. Carefully staged press conferences thus alternate with terse "no comments."

6. The theory and practice of deterrence is uniquely important to law-enforcement style regulation. The optimal level of law-enforcement activity for the achievement of policy goals is thus often difficult to determine. What appears to be a highly limited effort may produce as much impact as possible; incremental additions of regulatory resources will produce diminishing marginal returns. There will, on the other hand, also be many situations in which incremental additions can generate enormous returns.

Model IV: Contracting

The federal government is by far the largest purchaser of goods and services in the nation. In many markets, particularly including those for advanced armaments and some kinds of scientific research, it is a monopsonist of considerable power. As a result, an elaborate apparatus of legislation, procedures, and administration has grown up around governmental purchasing. This apparatus engages, in turn, in substantial regulatory activity, and the potential for additional regulation is high. The primary characteristics of regulation through contracting are these:[k]

1. Because the primary function of contracting remains the acquisition of goods and services or the supply of a subsidy, regulatory activities under contracting tend to be tangential or secondary activities, "added on" to the basic administrative function. Even when contracting-related regulation is important enough to merit creation of a separate and autonomous administrative structure, as in the Office of Civil Rights of HEW, those agencies occupy, relative to the central purchasing function, a rather passive staff—rather than line—position.

---

[k]The contracting model has been drawn primarily from: Walter Adams and William James Adams, "The Military-Industrial Complex: A Market Structure Analysis," 62, *American Economic Review Papers and Proceedings* (May, 1972), pp. 279-287; Harold Orlans, *Contracting for Atoms: A Study of Public Policy Issues Posed by the Atomic Energy Commission's Contracting for Research, Development, and Management Services* (Washington: The Brookings Institution), 1967; Don K. Price, *Government and Science: Their Dynamic Relation in American Democracy* (Oxford: Oxford University Press), 1954, Chapter III; and Larry Paul Ellsworth, "Defense Procurement: Everyone Feeds at the Trough," in Mark J. Green, ed., *The Monopoly Makers: Ralph Nader's Study Group Report on Regulation and Competition* (New York: Grossman Publishers), 1973, pp. 227-256.

In another syllogism, contracting often occurs without regulatory content, but this form of regulation is dependent on the maintenance of a high level of contracting activity.

2. If nothing else, the government is an informed buyer. Its legal—and often its administrative—ability to specify with great exactitude the items it wants to purchase, and to ascertain the extent to which those purchased meet its specifications, is constrained only by the inherent difficulties of measuring and evaluating purchases in the "softer" sectors of social services and professional performance. Sometimes, indeed, the government purchases things that do not yet even exist—as when it contracts, with detailed performance specifications, for new military hardware or educational training programs. Like law enforcement, contracting is highly discretionary, both in the sense of discretion over what will be contracted for and what the specifics of the contract will contain, and in the sense of who will receive contracts. For that reason, contracting has long been a primary focus of patronage and corruption—perhaps more so in state and local governments than at the national level, although not inconsiderably there. The creation of ever more complex rules and procedures to constrain administrative discretion in contracting—through requirements for competitive bidding, public notice, and so forth—appears to have generated an enormous volume of red tape with only limited practical impact.

3. The particular leverage of contracting as a regulatory device lies in its impact on considerations secondary to the intrinsic characteristics of the items purchased. Through contracting, the government affects employment discrimination, wage rates paid to construction workers, accounting practices of firms large and small, the allocation of time between teaching and research in university departments, and the survival chances of small businesses.

4. In certain instances, contracting relationships can be discouraging to potential entrants into a particular industry. Especially in the procurement of certain highly sophisticated forms of military hardware, it is often charged, the information and experience acquired by individual firms through past contracts, research and development work, and bid preparation give an important advantage to those already controlling a large share of the market. On the other hand, there have been numerous instances in which awareness of government intention to begin contracting for certain classes of goods or services has encouraged entry. Examples include private consultants and computerized educational techniques.

5. The preoccupation of legislators and public administrators with the fear of pecuniary scandals creates an emphasis on avoiding outright fraud—without appearing to reduce the incidence of scandals—to the exclusion of other goals of contracting. To a lesser extent, legislative oversight and public attention tend to concentrate on anomalies and exceptions, such as Senator Proxmire's annual burlesque on NSF appropriations.

6. Although government agencies have enormous discretion in creating and describing the contracts into which they have entered, once contracting is

underway the tools of enforcement are blunt and often self-defeating. The only sanctions available are generally those of termination or the assessment of financial penalties, which, if large enough to hurt, are functionally equivalent to termination. The government thus often develops a vested interest in not punishing contractors for non- or malfeasance, and looks the other way or even rewards them. As so often happens when formal sanctions are both stringent and inflexible, varieties of informal, extralegal bargaining between regulators and regulatees arise. Anyone who has ever participated in the government contracting process can attest that this bargaining provides regulations with considerable leverage and discretion. On the other hand, it creates personal ties and a community of interests between regulators and regulatees, often blurring the thin line between cooperation and collusion.

The Models and the Health Sector

The most convenient way to summarize the four models is to present them in tabular form. (see table 6-1). What is missing from that table is any explicit cognizance of how the models apply to the health sector. In some instances, the application is easy. Much of the work of the Food and Drug Administration, and of state and local agencies charged with administration of traditional public health codes, falls clearly into the law enforcement model. The licensure of health personnel remains almost a stereotype of licensure regulation at its worst, and seems, unfortunately to have been largely imitated by facilities licensure agencies.[19] Research grants and contracts under the National Institutes of Health, the National Institute of Mental Health, and the Health Resources Administration fit the contracting pattern, as do grants to operating agencies under categorical programs like those for community mental health centers or drug treatment programs. And nascent state rate-review commissions appear to have been more or less self-consciously patterned on the utility regulation model.[20]

Nonetheless, a number of prominent existing or proposed national health programs do not seem to fit any of the categories—and that very fact has significant implications, suggesting the absence of effective regulatory content. The much-discussed National Health Planning and Resources Development Act of 1974 (P.L. 93-641), for example, does strengthen certificate-of-need procedures, a form of licensing that has been notably ineffective at controlling supply, since the interests of providers are generally expansionary rather than restrictive.[21] Apart from certificate of need, however, the lofty aims of the act are not accompanied by regulatory teeth, other than the power to affect a small proportion of government contracting. P.L. 93-641, in other words, is hardly a regulatory statute at all.

Far more notable is the noncongruence of the two centrally important national health programs— Titles XVIII and XIX, Medicare and Medicaid—with any of the regulatory categories. Between them, the two programs account for more than two-thirds of total government health spending, but their system of "vendor payments" and service benefits, likely to be perpetuated under proposed forms of national health insurance, is basically inimical to regulatory action. Indeed, it appears to have been a conscious decision by legislators and executive-branch officials that the only way to ensure acquiescence of politically powerful providers, and therefore gain adoption of the programs at that outset, was to avoid creating even the appearance of interfering with provider prerogatives and autonomy.[22] Such regulation as was attempted in the initial legislation involved reliance on pitifully weak state licensing.

Over the ten-year history of the programs, cost escalation, combined with continued political reluctance to confront directly the prospect of regulation, have led Congress to add additional regulatory bits and pieces, involving elements of all four regulatory categories. Lacking coherence or systematic intent, they have had limited practical impact. They include more stringent definitions of allowable charges and other accounting conventions (utility regulation);[23] redoubled efforts to legislate against fraud and dishonesty in vendor billing and practices (law enforcement)—largely unaccompanied by enforcement efforts;[24] requirements that the Federal Life Safety Code be incorporated into state licensing criteria (licensing);[25] and the requirement of devices like utilization review and PSROs as conditions for the receipt of government payments.

The uncoordinated diversity of techniques reflects the ambivalence of policy makers towards effective regulation of providers, and it also creates the bureaucratic maze of rules and requirements that has generated so much hostility. Tacking regulation onto insurance-style financing might thus be described as a policy that, by attempting all kinds of regulation simultaneously, succeeds at none. Logically—as Congress is increasingly coming to realize—regulation must precede financing, rather than being the tail that attempts to wag the dog.

The most notorious of the vendor-payment programs, Medicaid, also illuminates another omission from the classification scheme. In some sense, intergovernmental grants-in-aid fall squarely into the contracting category. But in other ways they do not. The regulatees in that case are sovereign states that engage in regulation of their own. Many federal regulatory requirements are thus administered in a two-step process of contracting between federal and state governments and licensing or some other form of regulation by the states. In such an arrangement, "cooperative federalism" quickly degenerates into mutually antagonistic bureaucratic buck passing, in which each level of government resents the other's requirements while having little incentive to enforce its own.

The Models Compared

Although there is some value to a simple presentation of the four models of regulation, a comparison is far more important to policy choice.

Common Characteristics

As it is immediately apparent, table 6-1 contains no clues about how well the activities are performed and the functions fulfilled in each of the models. That characteristic has significant implications for the process of public policy debate, for the procedural and methodological content of this chapter, and for the particular question of alternative regulatory techniques for the health sector.

As a first approximation, it seems safe to say that anything attempted by government can be done well or done poorly. Although some contend that any government activity will, at a minimum, necessarily be somewhat less efficient than similar activities performed by the private sector, a not inconsiderable ideological bias underlies that argument. Yet the intrinsic fallibility of all human institutions is rarely given adequate shrift in policy debates. In order to sensibly evaluate alternative policy techniques it is necessary to compare degenerate form with degenerate form, effective form with effective form, and the relative likelihood of degeneration. This three-step process of comparison is far more realistic than the common terms of policy debate.

It is a central argument of this chapter that many of the shortcomings commonly attributed to utility regulation are characteristic of the degenerate forms of *all* types of regulation in the United States. As a result, they provide no basis for choosing between alternative regulatory forms, unless it can be demonstrated that there are good reasons to expect that some form is less likely to degenerate than others. Instead, the relevant choice is between the necessary evils associated with any kind of regulation (or, more generally, any kind of government intervention) and the necessary evils associated with existing markets. Actionable differences—between degenerate forms, or in the tendency to degenerate, or in the capabilities of nondegenerated techniques – are discussed later. Those characteristics with which we are likely to be stuck in the degenerate form of any kind of regulation are capture, conflict avoidance, life cycles and incrementalism and the absence of standards.

Capture. The single dominant theme in the radical-liberal critique of utility regulation has been the "capture" of regulatory bodies by the firms they are supposed to regulate.[26] In recent years, economists of differing political orientations have come to agree with this initially populist position. They have agreed that the primary effective function of utility regulation is the creation and maintenance of a closed cartel, administering cartel-level prices under the shield of government oversight.[27]

Even if the "capture" model provides an accurate description of behavior under utility regulation, it provides a similarly accurate model of the degenerate form of most of the other activities government undertakes, at least in those areas of policy in which business firms and professional individuals form part of the constituency. It is precisely Lowi's point that the Department of Agriculture is no less a captive of powerful farm interests than the Interstate Commerce Commission is of the railroads.[28] On a somewhat different tack, Mancur Olson's model of collective action, which provides a basic element of the capture theory espoused by many economists, applies to all situations in which relatively small, homogeneous groups receive, or seek to receive, a collective benefit from government, the costs of which are likely to be borne by the unorganized, heterogeneous population.[29] Olson's argument thus explains not only the Federal Communications Commission but also maritime subsidies, the conversion of the Arkansas River into a navigable waterway as far upstream as Tulsa, and large part of the Internal Revenue Code.

The other three models of regulation presented here are certainly no less subject to capture by interest groups. Licensing, as has already been noted, is dominated by interest groups, often through statutory provision. Academics often point at defense procurement through contracting as a particularly severe locus of "capture," as evidenced not only by the constant stream of retiring officers into executive positions in defense firms, but by the continued low-cost use of government-owned facilities by contractors and, in the extreme case, by the solicitude shown towards particular favorites such as Grumman or Lockheed.[30] Nonetheless, it was not DOD, but NIH, that was described as "the only pork barrel where the pigs decide who get the pork."[31]

The law-enforcement model might, at first glance, appear to be an exception, but if the mental image of homicide cases can be put aside for a moment, it is clear that there as well regulation is characterized by interchange of personnel between regulators and regulatees, heavy reliance by regulators on regulatees for information, and tendencies towards the development of more inclusively symbiotic relationships. It has often been pointed out, merely as an example, that food processors have a vested interest in stringent enforcement by the FDA—for the national brands, at least, it shifts costs onto the public purse while protecting producers from certain kinds of liability.[32]

More generally, the interests of special groups, especially producer groups, retain considerable legitimacy in both constitutional and political theory and the cultural values of citizens and government officials. The First Amendment right to petition for redress of grievances is a sacred underpinning of American administrative law and practice. The line between appropriate solicitude for private interests and outright capture is thus very fine and very thin. It should not be surprising that it is so frequently transgressed.[33]

Conflict Avoidance. Unhappy with the more conspiratorial undertones of the capture theory and the many empirical counterexamples, students of regulation have recently begun to develop a more sophisticated model of the behavior of utility-regulation agencies. George Hilton has provided the pungent name of "minimal squawk" for this theory.[34] It holds that members of utility-regulation commissions are motivated primarily by a desire to actively displease as few parties capable of making trouble for them as possible. Regulated firms are not the only constituents of this category; public groups, legislators, and especially the courts must also be propitiated. Regulators therefore make those decisions that can be expected to generate the least serious dissatisfactions by attempting to strike a balance or compromise among the demands of interested parties and by ritually observing all the procedural requirements necessary to avoid being overruled by the judiciary. The elaborate formal proceedings in which utility-regulation agencies engage have as a primary function, therefore, only that of protecting the rear from judicial intervention; the substantive content of decisions represents primarily a splitting of the difference between the demands of the parties at interest.[35]

More generically, the minimal-squawk theory might be translated into that of taking the path of least resistance. As such, it can be said to characterize bureaucratic behavior in general — if not much of the rest of human behavior. A pervasive characteristic of bureaucracy is the disproportion between punishment and reward: approved behavior often goes, if not unrecognized, at least unrewarded, and disapproved behavior generates expressions of disfavor if not more substantial sanctions. Playing it safe is frequently the more rational stragegy.

Thus prosecutors engaged in law enforcement in the criminal-justice system seek plea-bargained settlements because, in an overloaded and underfinanced criminal-justice system, the opprobrium attached to losing a trial is far greater than the rewards for winning one.[36] Similar behavior often characterizes law-enforcement agencies engaged in economic regulation. Better to settle for a consent decree than run the risk of being thrown out of court by a judge, or investing half the annual budget in a trial. Contracting officers go to elaborate lengths to preserve all appearances of fairness and impartiality while still managing to spread the rewards as broadly as possible among competing claimants; "splitting the difference," although perhaps hard to document, is pervasive there as well. Although licensing agencies are generally unable to split the difference in the binary decisions they are often forced to make, they have certainly shown reluctance to run afoul of the courts, and thus engage in ever more strenuous efforts to build both "objectivity" and "fairness" into their procedures.[1]

---

[1]For an extreme example, see Lawrence K. Altman, "State Officials Attribute Delay in Dr. Jacobson Case to Staff and Fund Limitations and Legal Maneuvers," *The New York Times,* April 28, 1975, 15:1.

Jerome Skolnick has suggested that, in a culture like that of the United States, adversary systems tend to degenerate into patterns of collusive cooperation. Impetus is provided both by cultural norms and organizational maintenance needs.[37] Since in some sense all government regulation is inherently adversary, Skolnick's theory suggests that it can therefore always be expected to degenerate into patterns of conflict avoidance. It might be added in passing that the degeneration of open conflict into tacit cooperation is characteristic of many parts of the private sector as well.

Life Cycles. A still older critique of utility regulation argues that regulatory agencies are subject to a life cycle in which initial enthusiasm is supplanted by middle-aged lassitude, and eventually by senescence.[38] Created in a burst of popular enthusiasm and indignation, the utility-regulation agency leaps blindly into the fray, its young and aggressive staff eager to fulfill the full implications of its statutory mandate. Resistance soon develops. The courts look askance on the agency's more aggressive or peremptory actions; affected firms and localities seek redress through congressional pressure; the general public and congressional appropriations committees soon lose interest. Retrenchment sets in; the agency becomes more cautious and slow to act. Disillusioned, the brightest and most aggressive young staff members leave (often to positions with regulated firms) and are replaced by individuals more sympathetic to the regulated industries. The final stage of this process—the ICC is everyone's favorite example—is the nadir of bureaucratic torpor. Bored timeservers ritualistically observe increasingly expanding, but increasingly meaningless, procedural rituals that have ever less and less to do with substantive policy.[39] But the life cycle need not be irreversible. Political changes, shifts in public opinion, or even the inspiration of a few idiosyncratic leaders can generate a revival. Interest is renewed, bright new staff are recruited, policy undergoes dramatic changes. Eventually, however, the aging process will again set in—the life cycle is not irreversible, but it is almost inevitable.

The major federal utility-regulation agencies, and many of those in the states, certainly seem to have undergone such cycles. The FCC, SEC, and FPC all seem to have experienced revivals in the 1960s after decades of relative lassitude. Some state agencies have similarly been revived, notably the insurance departments in New York and Pennsylvania. Nonetheless, the degenerative tendency of utility-regulation agencies to age badly is hardly limited to them. Again, it is a generic characteristic of bureaucratic administration. Anthony Downs' model of the "life cycle of bureaus,"[40] is the most detailed and elaborate explanation, but hardly the only one. Examples of the bureaucratic life cycle abound—indeed, it seems safe to say that the only exceptions are those agencies that never get off the ground in the first place (the centralized Drug Enforcement Agency being the most glaring recent example) or that are too young to have properly begun to age. In licensing, examples are provided by the Medicaid Office of New York City's Department of Health (now being revived) or generations of state liquor or liquor control authorities or the Office of Investigation of the Grains Division of the Department of Agriculture.[41] For law enforcement, no better example exists than the FBI, although the life cycle of the FDA bears important resemblances to a roller coaster.[42] Herbert Morton has documented the cyclical nature of activity under Walsh-Healy regulation of federal contracting,[43] and the Department of Defense, generally under congressional prodding, occasionally undergoes spasms of renewed energy in the enforcement of its contract provisions.

Incrementalism and the Absence of Standards. Since everyone agrees the one thing private firms do not do very well is plan, and since exhortations to develop systematic national policy are often contained in the statutory charters of utility-regulation agencies, another recurrent theme in the critique of utility regulation has been the continued pattern of ad hoc decision making, fragmented and often self-defeating policy formulation, and case-by-case adjudication.[44] Rare attempts to engage in more synoptic policy planning, through activities like the Federal Power Survey or the Special Study of the Securities Market, are pointed to both as examples of what should be and as rare exceptions.[45] Proposals for increased attention to planning and policy development appear in the conclusions of almost all studies of utility regulation.

The inability of utility regulation to plan, or even to act coherently, springs from two primary sources. The first is political. Even with relatively long terms for commissioners, regulatory agencies are only somewhat more immune than everyone else in Washington to the underlying quadrennial rhythm of life. The mandated partisan balance on most utility-regulation commissions and the ability of the president to appoint a commissioner means that, even in circumstances of relatively low turnover, changes in party control of the White House are often reflected before long in changes of regulatory policy. Congressman John Moss (D-Calif.) has recently suggested that the current wave of disillusionment with the effectiveness of federal regulatory agencies is not unrelated to six-and-a-half years of Republican control of the executive branch.[46]

Far more central to the absence of coherent policy planning, however, is the problem of standards. So generic is that problem to regulation of all kinds, and so relevant to the problems of the health sector, that it bears some discussion. Licensing, law enforcement, and in many instances contracting are equally subject to the problem of formulating clear and coherent standards of action. The problem is simply that, in many instances, no one knows enough. The FCC's "Fairness Doctrine" has been much ridiculed, but no one has been able to come up with an adequate substitute that both prevents abuses of monopoly power and avoids infringing on the First Amendment. There are similarly no meaningful, generally agreed-upon standards of moral character and fitness, or the "need" for a health facility, or the efficacy of a patent medicine, or whether or not the therapeutic advantages of a new drug outweigh its potential disadvantages, or whether a complex product of defense or atomic energy or biomedical research and development meets, on balance, contractual performance specifications.[47] In the regulatory arena, problems of standard setting are further complicated by the inability of consumers or the general public to make reasoned judgments about quality or usefulness—indeed, the very absence of adequate information or knowledge often provides much of the rationale for regulation in the first place.

I do not want to argue against the intrinsic desirability of standards setting, or to justify the failures of regulatory agencies in areas where standards setting has been avoided only from incompetence or sloth. But it is fair to say that the charge of incoherence and inadequate planning—of incrementalism in policy development—cannot be fairly laid against utility regulation, or all of regulation, alone. It is a pervasive characteristic of democratic government, true of the Department of State no less than the Civil Aeronautics Board.

Common Characteristics: Additional Comments. Two general themes underly the four common characteristics of the degenerate forms of all four regulatory models. The first is the pervasiveness of politics. Regulatory agencies are remarkably responsive to political tendencies and pressures.[48] Whether that is good or bad depends, of course, both on one's general perspective and on how one feels about the people holding power at any given time. If a body of systematic, objective knowledge, properly insulated from the political process were available, or if unregulated markets could function satisfactorily in all respects, regulatory agencies might be unnecessary. To the extent that those two alternatives are unrealistic, however, politicized regulation is probably the best we can do. The policy problem becomes one of controlling and managing politicization to meet the objectives of public policy, instead of frustrating them.

The second general characteristic might be described as the "wise-guy" effect. No matter how comprehensive or systematic a set of regulatory standards may be, some wise guy is going to think of a way to get around them. Regulation is always going to induce "distortions" in behavior, as individuals and firms prevented from doing what they wanted to do seek to get around the spirit but not the letter of regulation.[m]

To take such behavior as evidence of an inherent shortcoming of regulation is, however, to misread fundamental patterns of social behavior. To the extent that actions designed to evade a set of social norms without blatantly violating them are distortions, all kinds of social relationships are distorted; the only question is: who is doing the distorting? There is no a priori reason to believe

---

[m]The "wise-guy effect" is implicit in much of what Jaffe, "The Effective Limits of the Administrative Process: A Reevaluation," 67, *Harvard Law Review* (May 1954), p. 113, has to say about the "dynamism" of the private sector.

that distortions created by the exigencies of the market are any more socially beneficial that any others — nor any worse. The same reasoning applies to regulation-induced distortions. Their desirability or undesirability is a situational question, which can only be answered on a case-by-case basis.

Evaluative Criteria

If, as the preceding section suggests, the choice of regulatory technique may well consist of a choice among competing evils, it should still be possible, given some set of preferences, to opt for the least evil. There are systematic differences among regulatory techniques, some of which affect outcomes of the regulatory process.

Seven criteria have been chosen as the basis for that comparison. The first five have been adopted from those generally employed in discussion of industrial behavior and the impact of regulations on it. They are prices, efficiency, equity, quality, and progressiveness. Two additional criteria are also discussed. The first, administrative cost, is self-explanatory. What I call the *impact on social fabric*, which might be subtitled the "Titmuss effect," is not, but although it describes a complex phenomenon, it is relatively easily defined as the impact of a given set of political and administrative mechanisms on the quality of social relationships within the industry involved and in society as a whole.

Prices. Holding demand constant, the total public and private cost of health services is obviously a direct function of the level of prices. As noted earlier, much of the impetus for regulation in the health sector comes from the problem of total costs, especially those to the public sector, and the apparent appeal of utility regulation lies primarily in its direct focus on prices. The economic literature on the impact of regulation on prices in other sectors is abundant and confusing, leading, as the literature tends to do in economic questions of major public-policy significance, to no clear-cut conclusions. The safest generalization is that prices under utility regulation tend to fall somewhat below those that a pure cartel would administer, and somewhat above those that would be produced by a free market.[49]

The applicability of that experience to the health sector is similarly baffling. On the one hand, it is impossible to control hospital prices, or even sensibly tie them to costs, unless one has relatively standardized methods of cost accounting. The thrust towards regulation may finally be creating one for the hospital industry.[50] Regulatory lag might slow the pace, if not the magnitude, of price increases, which may be the best that can be hoped for. At current rates of inflation, health-care prices are increasing more than 10 percent a year.[51] One six-month delay in the growth rate could therefore produce aggregate savings of many billions of dollars.

More promisingly, it is fair to say that if anything (other than price control) has exercised a restraining effect on health-care prices in the last decade, it has been the sporadic attempts by Blue Cross to contend with hospitals on individual-price items.[52] Utility-regulation agencies might be expected to do no worse. Cost-conscious Blue Cross-Blue Shield plans have been able to constrain the market power of providers by forcing them into a duopolistic, zero-sum bargaining process. Utility regulation might act similarly. "Splitting the difference" between provider demands and consumer-presented alternatives might produce much lower rates of increase. Finally, utility regulation does have the virtue of its faults. Alone among regulatory devices, it does focus directly on prices, and if there is enough popular pressure, it is likely, at some point in its life cycle, to set prices lower than they would be in its absence.

On the other hand, price setting through utility regulation has certain shortcomings. First, health-care prices, particularly those in the hospital and nursing-home industry, have been expecially dominated by "pass-alongs." Health care, again, is a labor-intensive industry with few meaningful returns to capital per se. To the extent that utility regulation is able to control prices by constraining returns to capital, while permitting the passing along of generous returns to labor, it is likely to have little impact on health-care prices. Here the experience from other industries is unpromising. Returns to both labor and management in regulated industries tend to be higher than in unregulated firms.[n] Although desires to achieve high rates of return on capital provide incentives for the managers of public utilities to control labor costs, those incentives are largely lacking in the health industry, where revenues flow primarily to self-employed professionals and nonprofit institutions.

Second, to the extent that in the long run costs in the health-care industry can only be constrained by systematic reorganization,[o] utility regulation is unlikely to be of much help. Here again, the experience from other sectors suggests that the more common tendency of utility regulation is to freeze existing patterns of service and market structure rather than to rationalize them.[53]

In sum, then, although it is possible that utility regulation would have an impact on prices in the health sector, that impact is not likely to be very great. Utility regulation by itself might slightly moderate the rate of price increases, but is unlikely to limit prices any more severely than that.

---

[n]In April, 1975, average hourly earnings in "Transportation and Public Utilities"–a reasonable surrogate for the regulated sector of the economy–were $5.71, as opposed to $4.72 for "Manufacturing," and $4.44 for private industry as a whole. *Statistical Abstract of the United States,* 1975, pp. 366.

[o]It is interesting that such a reorganization is implicit in both "conservative" (emphasizing greater competition) and "radical" (emphasizing nationalization, community control, and deprofessionalization) critiques of the existing system.

The most notable regulatory thrust in the health sector in the past several years has been the development of certificate-of-need legislation and agencies. The rationale for this form of regulation is rooted in the belief that excessive capital expansion of the health industry, itself partially a result of government policy, notably the Hill-Burton Act, has had a significant role in the upwards spiral of prices, and that a licensing form of regulatory activity could at least rationalize future facilities construction.[p]

Even the most extreme estimate of the economic impact of the oversupply of health facilities puts the annual excess cost at $8 billion a year,[54] well under 10 percent of total health expenditures, and that figure has been hotly disputed.[55] More to the point, cost control through licensing suffers from the generic infirmities of that technique. It remains an essentially passive activity,[56] forced to rely on "objective" criteria only problematically related to public-policy objectives.[q] Although many certificate-of-need agencies are, in these early stages, dominated by administrations relatively unsympathetic to industry interests, there is no reason to expect that the life-cycle phenomenon has been permanently avoided; as public and governmental attention is captured by competing passing fancies, the more intense, full-time concerns of the industry may become more dominant.[57] As Clark Havighurst has noted, certificate-of-need regulation is likely to have the expected restrictive impact on entry even in those parts of the health sector where competition could have beneficial effects, as with health-maintenance organizations (HMOs) and, perhaps, skilled-nursing facilities.[58]

To the extent that facilities overbuilding creates a deadweight loss that must eventually be borne by consumers, then, certificate-of-need licensing can help control prices, although its ultimate impact will never be more than marginal. Whether those savings will counterbalance the increased costs of the regulatory process itself, let alone the possible increased prices resulting from restrictions on competition, remains to be seen.

Regulation through other forms of licensing, on the other hand, has clearly had an inflationary impact on prices. By controlling entry, and therefore supply, in markets for which demand is relatively unlimited, licensing can have little other effect.[59] That is not to say, however, that licensing must inevitably contribute to high prices. Two policy alternatives conceivable under licensure might

---

[p]On certificate-of-need regulation, see Havighurst, "Regulation of Health Facilities"; Harris S. Cohen, "Regulating Health Care Facilities: The Certificate of Need Process Re-Examined," X *Inquiry* (September 1973), pp. 3–9; William J. Bicknell and Diana Chapman Walsh, "Certificate of Need: The Massachusetts Experience," 292, *New England Journal of Medicine* (May 15, 1975), pp. 1054–1061; Eddie Correia, "Public Certification of Need for Health Facilities," 65, *American Journal of Public Health* (March 1975), pp. 260–265; and Lewin and Associates, *State and Regional Health Regulation,* Chapter IV.

[q]On the problem of standards in certificate-of-need regulation, see Lewin and Associates, *State and Regional Health Regulation* pp. 4–100.

well have a moderating impact. The first would be to simply alter the role of licensing agencies from restrictive to expansionary, by encouraging alternative career paths to eligibility standards for individual professionals (as for American-born students forced to attend foreign medical schools) or by sanctioning unconventional administrative or organizational arrangements for the delivery of services. Using licensing in this way would raise questions about ensuring the quality of services, but appropriate means of doing so might well be found.

A more potent impact on prices might result from efforts to create some awareness by physicians of the economic impacts of their behavior on health-care costs.[r] Since the medical schools have failed to leap into this breach, licensing authorities might create incentives for them by requiring their graduates to demonstrate a minimal level of awareness of the issues involved. On balance, nonetheless, licensing offers little hope for controlling prices.

To the extent that outright fraud or abuse play a part in inflating the costs of health care, regulation through law enforcement does offer some promise for having an impact on price. Fraud probably does play a larger role in the nation's total health-care bill than most students of health services would be eager to admit,[60] and continued movement towards national health insurance can only exacerbate the existing imbalance in which individual patients have little incentive to keep an eye on provider behavior (and may often enter into collusive arrangements with providers), while the victim is an impersonal, faceless third party. Moreover, law enforcement against health-care fraud contains some elements that conduce to the prevention of administrative degeneration. Those engaged in prohibited activity are highly visible, not in need of the money, and unlikely objects for public sympathy. One imagines it is not hard to get a jury to convict for Medicaid fraud. Resource-allocation decisions are relatively simple, since each dollar spent in this way on law enforcement is likely to generate several in revenues, up to a relatively high point.

Still and all, there is no imaginable way in which directly dishonest behavior can be made to account for more than a small fraction of total health-care expenditures. Even if the nursing-home industry, honestly run homes are expensive, and the issue is more one of enforcing standards than controlling prices; exorbitant profits come directly out of the well-being of the patients.[s] So although some regulatory effort through law enforcement is essential, and will become more so, it will hardly provide a panacea.

The notion that government regulation through standards setting and enforcement is inflationary seems to have replaced creeping socialism as the

---

[r]Fuchs emphasizes behavioral changes by physicians as essential to cost control without, however, suggesting any mechanisms for achieving them. Cf. *Who Shall Live?* pp. 103–104.

[s]For a more extended discussion, see Vladeck, "Public Utility Regulation and the Nursing Homes."

favorite battle cry of conservative corporate interests.[61] Obviously, if inferior goods are banned from the marketplace, their replacements will be more expensive; *changes* in regulations create compliance costs that may well exceed the short-run benefits of the regulation; and there have undoubtedly been many unwise, irrational, and excessively costly regulations. But no matter how much economists may quibble about the valuation of a human life, the very existence of most such regulations in a putatively democratic society can only be assumed to be evidence of a social decision that the increased costs to consumers are worth it.

The relationship of contracting to cost control is more paradoxical. On the one hand, if there is any conclusion to be drawn from the experience with contracting in other sectors, it is that it drives costs *up*.[62] Much of the reimbursement for contractors providing goods and services to the government is on a cost-plus basis, which provides little incentive for cost control. Contracting officers themselves, as well as the line officials who request purchases, have incentive to "gold-plate" specifications, adding expensive but only marginally useful requirements, thus increasing costs. And the incentive for sellers to "buy in" to contracts by deliberately misestimating on the low side, when combined with the limited effectiveness of sanctions against overruns, hardly contributes to price minimization.[63]

Those instances in which contracting can be effected through competitive bidding, on the other hand, do offer opportunities for substantial leverage over prices, in a way that should be particularly pleasing to economists. Although the government has as yet shown very little desire to do so, it would certainly be possible under national health insurance, and even under more limited programs such as Medicare, to purchase certain kinds of services in some areas through variants of competitive bidding.[t] Again, quality control might present a serious problem, but opportunities exist for creative policy making.

Contracting is highly subject to degeneration, perhaps more so than any other form of regulation. Put another way, it is a powerful instrument, but one prone to falling into disuse. Given the unwieldiness of termination as a sanction in health services, only an aggressive agency confident of fairly mobilized public support is likely to accomplish much in terms of price control through contracting. Tendencies to "rationalization" of the health-care system through the elimination of duplication in facilities and more equitable distribution of providers will only exacerbate that weakness, and further limit the ability of government to regulate health services through contracting.

---

[t]For an ingenious proposal, see Harold Hinderer, "Reimbursement: Past, Present, and Future," in Graduate Program in Hospital Administration and Center for Health Administration Studies, Graduate School of Business, University of Chicago, *Public Control and Hospital Operations,* Proceedings of the Fourteenth Annual Symposium on Hospital Affairs, May, 1972 (Chicago: Graduate Program), 1972.

Efficiency. Implicitly or explicitly, the principal evaluative criterion used by many economists in considering utility regulation is that of allocative efficiency. For all its shortcomings as a criterion, there can be little argument with the contention that, all other things being equal, a more allocatively efficient solution is to be preferred to a less allocatively efficient one. Although all other things are not equal, those inequalities are perhaps best dealt with in terms of the other criteria discussed here.

In a theoretically perfect market, the price system ensures attainment of optimal allocative efficiency. By its administrative manipulation of prices, therefore, utility regulation, according to the most common single indictment, removes incentives to the efficient use of resources and, indeed, often rewards inefficiencies. To the extent that the distortions created by higher or lower-than-market prices are not compensated for by countervailing social advantages or benefits, utility regulation thus creates a deadweight loss to society.[64]

Those losses, of course, exist only in comparison to the presumed market that would prevail in the absence of utility regulation. Although such markets might, conceivably, be restored to some industries currently subject to utility regulation—air transportation is probably the best example[65]—the notion that they might ever exist, or be somehow created, in the health sector is a pipe dream. Consumer demand for health services bears almost no resemblance to that in a classical Marshallian model, nor are the exclusionary effects of a market system on low-income consumers any longer tolerable in the provision of health care in advanced societies. More to the point, prices in the health sector are now, and have long been, almost purely administered prices.

On the other hand, utility regulation offers few positive incentives for efficient resource use. The existence of a detailed rate structure, alterations in which can only be achieved through difficult administrative proceedings, attaches costs to innovation and experimentation. Although voluntary hospitals are not subject to the pure form of the "Averch-Johnson" effect, a positive incentive to inefficiency through overcapitalization,[66] the absence of a fixed rate of return on a rate base does not imply that administrators are uninterested in maximizing gross costs.[67] In short, a system of utility regulation in the health industry is unlikely to encourage substantial improvements along the currently dismal dimension of allocative efficiency.

The extent of licensing that already pervades the health sector is often pointed to as a major source of inefficiency. By imposing severe restrictions on the use of the most expensive factor of production—professional and semi-professional manpower—it prevents individual facilities from combining manpower in the most effective way. State-by-state licensing of medical personnel creates a significant degree of artificial factor immobility, with consequent allocative distortions. This problem is likely to be rendered more severe by the increasing rate of licensure for very narrowly defined paraprofessional and semiprofessional occupations, with each state having its own classifications, definitions, and procedures. The restrictions on entry created by licensing often have inefficient allocative consequences.[68]

Yet it is not clear that any of the proposed solutions to these problems offer a realistic chance for improvement. One reform proposal, in particular, subsumes most of the others. That is the notion of institutional licensure, which would shift the locus of license holding from individuals to health facilities, which would then be free to employ personnel in whatever way they wished, and would thus presumably be able to make more efficient use of manpower.[69] Institutional licensure suffers two serious shortcomings. The first is that occupational licenses are not the only barriers to efficient manpower use. The licensure structure of a hospital or other health facility both reflects and is reflected in a complex set of status hierarchies, power distributions, and subcultural norms, which may have a larger impact on manpower use than anything on the statute books. Increased unionization of hospital employees is also likely to have a significant impact; collective bargaining creates its own barriers to administrative discretion in personnel assignments. Although superimposition of collective bargaining agreements on a complex system of licensure may have particularly restrictive implications—as it appears to have had in the public sector—elimination of individual licensure will not completely remove the problem.

The second shortcoming of institutional licensure has more direct policy implications. Licensing is a balky regulatory tool because the available range of sanctions is so limited. Even when the affected transgressor is only an individual, regulatory authorities are particularly loath to revoke licenses because of the magnitude of the punishment; but there are few intermediate enforcement steps available. It is almost inconceivable that a state or federal agency responsible for institutional licensure would revoke the license of a community's single hospital, or a facility on which influential citizens—or ghetto residents—are especially reliant, on grounds of simple inefficiency. When the supply of available facilities falls short of needs in a more general market—as Thomas's study of nursing homes in New York demonstrates[70]—regulatory authorities are unwilling to revoke any licenses. Regulation through licensing is thus rendered meaningless.

As already discussed, the allocative inefficiency created by the excessive building and duplication of facilities has been made subject to certificate of need regulation. However, the reliance of licensing authorities on the development of objective criteria would appear to limit the potential net efficiency effect of certificates of need, at least in the short run. Except in the most glaring instances (such as open-heart surgery) of inefficient duplication, no one really knows just how much is enough, and errors on the side of undersupply are just as inefficient as those on the side of oversupply.

If reforms in licensing regulation can be expected to have little impact on allocative efficiency, and extensions of existing licensing regulation through the recognition of still more narrowly defined categories of personnel can only make the situation worse, law enforcement is likely to do little good either, although its negative impact on efficiency is probably overstated. Law enforcement has little ability to compel affirmative behavior of any kind, and no one has yet devised a way of formulating prohibitions against waste, inefficiency, or stupidity. Although in certain instances law enforcement can create a "crime tariff," with consequent allocation distortions,[71] the evolutionary liberalization of social mores has effectively eliminated most such tariffs in the health sector—the legalization of abortion constituting the most significant recent example. Although the regulation of health, purity, and safety standards through law enforcement may induce some economically inefficient behavior in individual firms, it is hard to believe that the total social effect is inefficient in the aggregate.

Contracting is another matter. Indeed, of all the regulatory techniques considered here, it alone has the potential of creating incentives for efficiency. The extreme case arises in situations in which competitive bidding would be possible; so long as there were adequate administrative energy and commitment to avoidance of the disfunctions that can result from competition, the quasi-automatic impact of competition could have beneficial results.[72] Even in single-source contracting, however, there is considerable latitude for efficiency incentives. Contracts can be negotiated with a fixed fee, or a sliding-fee scale based on cost performance, or more specific incentives related to particular activities or obligations under the contract. "Incentive reimbursement" by a single buyer, such as Blue Cross, for hospital services is an almost pure form of attempted efficiency inducement through contracting regulation.[u] Although the early experience with incentive reimbursement has been disappointing, its failures appear to result from the conceptual shortcomings of the particular schemes, rather than from the basic idea of introducing efficiency incentives into a contrasting relationship. There is no logical reason, moreover, why the idea of incentive reimbursement could not be extended to physician services, especially to physicians practicing in groups—in essence, that is the economic intrarule for HMO's, and, one suspects, the source of their popularity among economists.[73]

Equity. Traditionally, the criterion of equity is operationally defined in policy analysis as the anticipated impact of a proposal on the distribution of income. That criterion is too limited for a discussion of the health sector. Eschewing the welfare economists' fiction that all psychic and sociopolitical costs and benefits can be treated under the rubric of "income," income-distribution effects are narrowly construed here to encompass only pecuniary rewards and deprivations

---

[u]On incentive reimbursement, cf. Fuchs, *Who Shall Live?*, pp. 100–102; Richard A. Elnicki, "SSA-Connecticut Hospital Incentive Reimbursement Experiment Cost Evaluation," XII, *Inquiry* (March 1975), pp. 47–58; Hinderer, "Reimbursement: Past, Present, and Future."

differentially affecting different *income* groups. Far more significant to health policy is the distribution of access to care among social groups distinguished from one another on criteria other than income. Policies seeking to improve that access within given provider institutions or networks are defined here as *cross-subsidization,* in the sense not of income transfers per se, but rather of the provision of intrinsically uneconomic services (which must of course create some kind of disbenefit for those who do not use them). Economists might not recognize the validity of this distinction, but the political meaningfulness is clear. The regulatory requirement that airline X provide service between small town Y and congressional district Z is politically a very different phenomenon from one that requires middle-income coach passengers to subsidize upper income first-class travelers, or vice versa. To the extent that health care is a right, the criterion of distributive justice—of equity—demands nonincome-related cross-subsidization.

The one thing utility regulation is particularly good at is the attainment of more equitable outcomes through cross-subsidization.[74] Users of residential telephone service, airline or rail transportation to smaller or isolated cities, and public-service or religious programming on television and radio all benefit from the power of utility regulation to compel the provision of uneconomic services in exchange for the granting of franchises and the right to charge higher prices to other customers. This is not to say, of course, that all cross-subsidization steals from the service rich to give to the service poor; under degenerative conditions, or in the absence of adequate theoretical or empirical knowledge, cross-subsidization can have undesirable effects.

Given the pervasiveness of cross-subsidization already prevailing in the health industry, the ineluctable necessity to continue it in some form for certain classes of patients who can never conceivably afford services to which society thinks them entitled, and the underlying truth that decisions about cross-subsidization of this kind involve the most basic dimensions of social choice, the appeal of utility regulation to those in the health-care industry is obvious. Direct subsidization of specified services is not an attractive alternative; there are just too many, with too many variable characteristics, serving too many variable patients. Moreover, direct subsidization tends to lead to an identification of its beneficiaries as charity cases or otherwise the objects of some special attention, creating the danger of a two-class or multiclass system of health care.

Licensing, as it now exists, certainly creates a transfer of income from non-license holders to licensees. It has even been argued that the principal economic effect of licensing in industries like television is the creation of wealth in the form of the capitalized value of licenses.[75] On the other hand, there appears to be growing sentiment for use of the licensing mechanism in order to create the cross-subsidization required in the health sector without incurring the disadvantages of utility regulation. Thus it has been proposed that the existing system of hospital licensure be replaced by a system of health-care franchises, in which the right to operate a facility would be granted only on the condition that a comprehensive set of services, including some that would not otherwise be provided by the private sector, be made available in adequate quantity for an entire geographic area.[v]

Such a franchising system would appear to avoid the danger of allocative distortions inherent in utility regulation price-setting while retaining the advantages of regulating the distribution of services. So long as the letter and spirit of the franchises were observed far more strictly than the implicit conditions of much contemporary licensing, such a policy would appear to have obvious benefits. On the other hand, the reinforcement through franchising of the tendency towards natural monopoly would raise the question of whether those possessing such enormous discretionary market power should be permitted to go largely unsupervised, since the incentives for efficiency and equity of treatment inherent in franchising (although there may be no *dis*incentives, as there can be in utility regulation) are highly limited. Historically, franchising has often been supplanted by utility regulation, since the potential for abuse of market power is so great, and the tendency of licensing to degenerate is so marked. Given the importance of health services, it is hard to imagine that a similar supplanting would not—or should not—develop.

As has been seen over and over again with the regulatory implications of law enforcement, the ability to deter prohibited behavior is largely unmatched by the ability to compel affirmative behavior. Since considerations of equity sometimes involve malfeasance and sometimes nonfeasance, the applicability of law-enforcement regulation to equity problems in the health sector will be highly variable. The enforcement of antidiscrimination statutes by the Office of Civil Rights of HEW has been far more effective than efforts to ensure that Hill-Burton-funded hospitals devote at least 5 percent of their services to charity.[76] Moreover, because income redistribution generally requires affirmative behavior of some sort, law-enforcement regulation is unlikely to have very much impact.

Direct-government contracting for the provision of services to groups or individuals who have equitable right to them but would not otherwise receive them is, of course, largely equivalent to subsidization through direct-service programs, with all the advantages and disadvantages inherent in that process. On the other hand, although it is relatively easy to write requirements for equitable distribution or availability into more general contracts, such as those that would necessarily arise under parts of national health insurance, it is a more difficult matter to see that those contractual requirements are carried out. Given the relative political status of those whose health needs would be subsidized,

---

[v]This is basically the proposal articulated by Anne Somers in "Regulation of Hospitals," pp. 79–81.

inadequate enforcement would be a perpetual problem—as it has been with the Hill-Burton 5 percent requirement. Cross-subsidization through a price system, as prevails under utility regulation, is more nearly self-enforcing than mandated cross-subsidization under contracting, and thus much less likely to be affected by administrative degeneration. To the extent that the costs of subsidizing certain groups are more equitably borne through government assumption of costs rather than subsidization by other classes of consumers, contracting has important advantages. The question of which method is to be preferred hinges largely on one's preferences about who should be paying for what.

Contracting has other implications for income distribution. It is difficult to lose money in the performance of a government contract, probably far more difficult than in the provision of services under utility regulation. The very existence of wide-scale contracting tends to encourage the entry of profit-seeking firms. The practice of contracting can, in other words, create returns to capital where none previously existed. To the extent one believes that the health sector is already overcapitalized, contracting thus has clear disadvantages, since the ability to attract capital might outweigh the distributive consequences, unless combined with a ban on the award of contracts to proprietary institutions, a constitutionally dubious idea.

Quality. Recent theoretical work has suggested that, under monopoly conditions, utility regulation may cope more effectively with quality-price trade-offs than unregulated markets.[77] Reality did not await theoretical developments. Quality of service is so important in the health sector, and so difficult for consumers to assess, that regulatory activity has long been considered unavoidable. Indeed, quality-based regulation in the health sector was politically acceptable long before any other kind, and continues to be a concern of almost everyone with an interest in health policy, regardless of their views on regulation of other aspects of the industry's performance.

Quality regulation through utility regulation suffers, however, from the problem of standards.[78] Utility regulation can be quite effective at enforcing quality standards when reasonable, quantitative criteria exist. It is relatively easy to define "on-time arrival" in the transportation industry, or proportion of pay phones out of service, for example.[79] Defining quality in health services is far more difficult. Existing standards tend to rely heavily on statistical artifacts that reflect existing patterns of service far more accurately than any sense of what might be desirable in the abstract.

In the last decade, Congress has acted as though it perceived the problem of health-sector costs as one of quality. Techniques like utilization review and PSROs, whatever their benefits in improved quality, will likely have little impact on total expenditures for personal-health care. If costs are indeed the problem, it would probably be far better to attempt to control them directly, and to treat quality control as a separate issue of inherently enormous intellectual complexity.[80]

Alternatively, one might argue that, to the still considerable extent that the practice of medicine is (and perhaps should continue to be) more art than science, quality is best maintained through ensuring the quality of practitioners, and then leaving them to the more or less free exercise of their professional judgment. In other words, if one doubts the ability of regulators and their associated computers to develop meaningful, general, quantitative standards that will account for a broad enough range of problems—and if one perhaps doubts as well the desirability of such standards—attention obviously turns to the process of licensing. If systematic provision could be made for periodic relicensure, continuing education, and the enforcement of sanctions on those who violate the basic precepts of the profession, licensing could probably accomplish as much in terms of quality regulation as is likely to be accomplished, at least in the foreseeable future. This licensing, it should be noted, would necessarily be personal and not institutional, since it is impossible to lodge responsibility in an institution.

Quality regulation through law enforcement suffers from the same difficulties as regulation through utility regulation with the problem of standards. To the extent that appropriate standards can be identified, as in the processing of canned and frozen foods, law enforcement can be extremely effective. But when judgment is necessarily more subjective and less precise, there is little that law enforcement can do.

The problems of imprecise, subjective judgment are often surmounted in contracting agencies through the device of peer review. As opposed to licensing, the regulation of quality through contracting with peer review has the significant advantage of applying to prospective as well as retrospective behavior. It has, however, the significant disadvantage of being considerably more time consuming and cumbersome, and of demanding the energies of just those individuals whose time is most valuable (and expensive). Since requirements for licensing can, of course, always be written into contracts, some dual system of mandatory licensing plus peer review on a sample or exceptions basis may provide the most effective possible form of quality control in those situations where precise quantitative standards are unavailable.

Progressiveness. Although the most systematic consideration of the subject concludes with a judgement that the evidence is equivocal, utility regulation has often been criticized for impeding technological innovation.[81] The putative tendency of utility regulation to impair technological change has, similarly, been offered as a reason for opposing its adoption in the health sector.[82] Yet, although the public perception of technological advance in health care as an unmitigated boon appears not to have changed, some knowledgeable individuals are beginning to question the desirability of the rapid and uncontrolled diffusion of new techniques, procedures, and equipment. Technological change has clearly been a major contributor to the escalation of health-care costs, although its impact on gross measures of population health—such as mortality or morbidity rates—appears to have been surprisingly slight.[83]

The tendency of utility regulation to delay change without preventing it altogether acquires a certain attractiveness when applied to the health sector. Yet much the same can be said of other regulatory techniques. In general, it can safely be said that all forms of regulation, with the possible exception of contracting, impede technological change. Contracting can actually promote such change, either by developing contractual specifications for beyond-the-state-of-the-art goods or services, or by permitting subsidization of research, development, and testing in the course of providing some good or service, or by merely providing the kinds of incentives for economic efficiency discussed above. On the other hand, to the extent that contracting specifies in detail the processes or methods through which contractual aims will be met, it can have a retarding effect on technological development. The imagination of contracting authorities is often limited, thus causing them to frown unproductively on the radically new and untried while rewarding conservatism and tradition.

The challenge to public policy, of course, is to develop mechanisms that will encourage "desirable" new technologies while discouraging "undesirable" ones. The debate over the impact of the Kefauver Drug Amendments notwithstanding, it probably makes little difference, at this stage in scientific and sociopolitical development, what mechanism is chosen, so long as there is one. Whether the form is a quasi-judicial utility-regulation or licensing body, a hierarchial standards-setting agency charged with law enforcement, or independent experts in an advisory relationship to contracting agencies, regulators will have to make informed guesses in a process necessarily slower, but safer, than that of the free market.

Administrative Cost. Although any systematic cost-benefit comparison includes the overhead costs of program administration, and although these should be considered for purposes of evaluating regulation as well, there is another, more important reason for including administrative cost as an evaluative criterion. As a rough rule of thumb, it seems safe to argue that the higher the administrative cost inherent in any policy alternative, the more susceptible that mechanism is to degeneration. Relatively self-enforcing policies have the advantage of needing no great commitment of political will or budgetary outlay to accomplish their goals. Policies requiring more costly and complex administrative activities are far more likely to be subject to passing political whims, to undergo cyclical expansions and contractions of effort, and to suffer from chronic subacute budgetary starvation. Since any policy is only as good as the effort with which it is administered, policy techniques that are intrinsically expensive or difficult create greater dangers of policy failure.[w]

---

[w]For a summary of the issues in the debate, see Fuchs, *Who Shall Live?*, pp. 115–119.

None of the regulatory models discussed here comes near to being self-enforcing. All are bulky and complex. But they do vary considerably in the size and complexity of the administrative apparatus necessary to carry them out. Utility regulation is far and away the most costly. Total costs for the regulatory process itself have been estimated to approach $1 billion a year at the federal level alone.[84] That amount is small relative to the magnitude of economic activity involved, but inferentially it has much to do with the chronic problems of understaffing and administrative lethargy in utility-regulation agencies.

Licensing is a considerably smaller industry, at least partially because the use of objective measures of performance conduces to more automatic and easier administrative practices than detailed case-by-case adjudication in adversary proceedings. Upgrading licensing to provide for continuing education and re-licensure would add considerably to complexity and costs, although it is unlikely that the problem would grow to be as severe as it is in utility regulation. One way of minimizing administrative cumbersomeness and cost, and controlling tendencies to degeneration, would be to adopt a system of centrally managed national licensing.

Because of the impact of deterrence, the resources necessary for successful law enforcement are somewhat more variable, depending heavily on the nature of the sanctions available and the acceptance by regulatees of the values and principles embodied in the standards being enforced.[85] Although there is always at least one dissenter at a hanging,[x] behavioral standards that reflect widely shared values impose considerably smaller administrative costs for law enforcement than those that embody more esoteric, narrowly held or unpopular prohibitions. These abstract considerations notwithstanding, the record of law enforcement in many areas of the health sector has been relatively impressive, and in others, most notably those programs involving vendor payments that have fallen between the three stools of licensing, contracting, and law enforcement, the experience has been nothing less than appalling. The Medicaid experience would suggest that at least in certain parts of the health sector, the power of moral standards and behavioral deterrence is distressingly low, requiring in turn especially vigilant law-enforcement activities that are unlikely to always prevail.

The costs of contracting administration are similarly variable, but there the variation results more from the problem of formulating standards than from that of gaining acceptance for them. When the government as buyer has a relatively clear idea of what it wants and can specify those desires in adequately precise terms, contracting administration can be relatively straightforward and simple. More complicated or ill-defined products, on the other hand, can require an almost literally infinite amount of administrative resources. When the government

---

[x]This felicitous phrase is of course stolen from E.E. Schattschneider, *The Semisovereign People: A Realist's View of Democracy* (New York: Holt, Rinehart and Winston), 1960, p. 24.

wants to buy aspirin, in other words, contracting is an easy process. When it wants to require affirmative action towards equal-employment opportunity, that is another matter.

Impact on Social Fabric. In his remarkable book, *The Gift Relationship: From Human Blood to Social Policy,* Richard Titmuss suggested that most evaluation of public policies is far too narrowly drawn. Policy is not merely a set of means for the attainment of a defined end; it also frequently has important implications for the ways in which people think, feel, and act towards one another. There is thus a kind of ripple effect, in which the content of an individual policy spreads out to affect the quality of social relationships everywhere in society.[86]

Because of the perceived importance of health services to modern life, the ways in which those services work and attempts at changing those ways are likely to have an effect outside the narrow sphere of the individual hospital or physician's office. Here, perhaps, lies the most trenchant basis for the rejection of free-market relationships in health care. The reduction of life and death to a set of commodities, bought and sold on the open market, involves the dehumanization and desocialization of caring, which many of us are not prepared to accept. Yet if that argument is relied upon to justify regulation of various aspects of the health sector, it is surely necessary to examine the expected impact of regulation on broader patterns of social life.

Utility Regulation is often described as suffering from "overjudicialization."[87] Like many blanket epithets, that has its limitation, but for regulatory proceedings in which the property rights involved are those of the owners or controllers of property, and in which the public interest in elaborate due-process guarantees is severely limited, the promotion of overjudicialization is hardly desirable. Most notable, in terms of "Titmuss effect," is the exclusionary impact on consumers and others significantly affected by the process.[88] As soon as something becomes sufficiently legalistic, complicated, and expensive, many who might otherwise have a legitimate interest are excluded, with important consequences for alienation and the quality of justice in public life.

The licensing of individuals has a very different kind of Titmuss effect. By conferring what is in essence a property right, it distributes status, prestige, and, often, self-esteem to license holders. When that distribution systematically favors those who already control a disproportionate share of society's resources, it exacerbates inequalities of power and status and the injustices and social tensions that go along with those inequalities.[89] When it creates prestige and property for those who formerly did not have any, however, its social consequences can be highly desirable. Whatever else one might say or feel about programs for the licensing of health sector paraprofessionals, they have created for many individuals, large numbers of whom are from minority groups, a sense of dignity and pride in their work they had never before been able to feel.[90] Institutional licensing, on the other hand, can only accelerate the social process of conferring

145

power and responsibility on institutions, rather than individuals. As a result, it would accelerate the too-potent trends to depersonalization, dehumanization, and diffusion of individual responsibility in modern society.

Law-enforcement activities have similarly variable Titmuss effects. Law enforcement works best when everyone obeys the law; it breaks down completely when no one does. That statement implies the need for some humility on the part of those who would attempt to study public policies in any kind of vacuum. To the extent that democratically determined standards of conduct are commonly evaded by any sizable number of persons (an operational definition of *sizable* would be: a lot more than law-enforcement agencies are able to catch), efforts at regulation are palliatives for a potentially fatal deterioration of the social fabric.

The creation and enforcement of contractual relationships, on the other hand, is likely to do far more good for the quality of social relationships than harm. Ours is a society based on the sanctity of covenants and the value of mutual reciprocity and respect. Contracting relationships reinforce those values— as do efforts to enforce contractual provisions. By definition, a *contract* identifies a community of interest, and the operative word is "community." On the other hand, there is often a community of interest between government officials and private firms or individuals to conspire against the public good − to engage in official corruption. Since corrupt contracts are by definition not legitimate ones, the prevention of corruption in contracting is thus a highly necessary and useful social activity, and the degeneration of contracting into corruption vitiates whatever useful social purposes it might have.

Comparative Characteristics: A Summary

The comparisons of the four models of regulation made in the preceding pages are summarized in table 6-2. As might have been expected, none of the four models is clearly preferable on a majority of the significant dimensions. Moreover, there are many evaluative criteria along which none of the models is clearly preferable. The most notable of these is the ability to control prices.

The entries in table 6-2 can be interpreted in two ways. First, they are, admittedly, often subjective generalizations based primarily on experiences in other sectors. Scholars of regulation might well disagree with the content of any particular entry, although every effort was made to be as reasoned and thorough as possible in incorporating existing knowledge about regulation. On the other hand, each of the cells also contains a behavioral prediction about the ways in which regulation in the health sector might be expected to work along each of the evaluative dimensions. The accuracy of those predictions can, of course, only be judged empirically.

Table 6-2
Summary of Comparisons of Regulatory Models

Criteria

Model	Prices	Efficiency	Equity	Quality	Progressiveness	Administrative Cost	"Titmuss Effect"
I. Utility Regulation	Might moderate rate of price increase	Negative; destroys allocative function of prices	Cross-subsidization powerful tool for achieving greater equity	Problem of standards	Impedes technological change	Considerable; creating strong tendency to degeneration	Overjudicialized protection of property rights
II. Licensing	Certificate of need as likely to increase prices as reduce them; licensing professionals inflationary unless cost consciousness added	Certificate of need could help; occupational licensure can hurt	Possibly inequitable returns to license holders; franchising a limited alternative	With continuing education and meaningful relicensure—excellent	Impedes technological change	Relatively small	Creates social prestige and power, for either advantaged or disadvantaged groups
III. Law Enforcement	Reduces dishonesty; produced cost only; impact therefore marginal	Marginal impact	Limited ability to compel affirmative behavior	Problem of standards	Impedes technological change	Depends on acceptance of standards by regulatees; can be very high	Depends on acceptance of standards by regulatees
IV. Contracting	Highly variable; reductions possible when competition is feasible	Can create efficiency incentives	Creates returns to capital, but can compel cross-subsidization	Peer review effective but costly; does permit prospective judgment	May encourage or impede technological change	Varies with nature of product; highly susceptible to corruption	Reciprocal contractual relationships have positive effects, but corruption often a problem

More immediately, however, the policy-relevant question, espcially in light of the seeming equivocalness of the evaluations summarized in table 6-2 is: so what? What do we do now? Although this chapter avoids drawing any hard and fast conclusions about "correct" courses of action, there are some summary generalizations possible that have implications for the process of policy choice and the identification of "better" policies.

Conclusions

The Problem of Limits

All government action is partial, self-limiting, and less than "synoptic." Perfect, comprehensive, self-enforcing policy is a chimera. Informed policy must thus be grounded in a recognition of the limits inherent in realistic alternatives. Incrementalist approaches, either in theory or practice, are particularly inappropriate for the exploration of those limits. Experience cumulates too slowly; and the world refuses to stand still while incremental testing takes place, thus limiting the value of constrained experience.[91] Although the notion of synoptic policy making implies an unrealistic sense of optimization, a more pragmatic method involving the kinds of comparisons undertaken here has obvious advantages. At least it can be suggested that the achievement of a specific goal through one technique is likely to be less costly than it would be through another, or that technique X will achieve objective J only to the extent that condition Z holds. The technique of "multiple, simultaneous comparisons," as opposed to "limited successive comparisons," permits judgments as to the *relative* advantages and disadvantages of several alternatives *and* the existing state of affairs.

Fortunately, the real world does not insist that individual policies conform to any abstract model. One can pick and choose various features of different alternatives—to the extent that their limits do not overlap. Congress has certainly shown no aversion to eclecticism in the framing of legislation, and a delineation of the inherent limitations of alternative techniques can help prevent eclecticism from sinking into a maze of self-contradictory half-measures.

Thus, in terms of the goal of quality control, for example, it is possible to combine licensing techniques with peer-review procedures of the kind often employed under contracting policies. The still further addition of an elaborate set of penalties for nonconformance, on the other hand, is unlikely to provide substantial additional benefit, and may be counterproductive to the extent it violates the norms of the community with which the government is contracting.

To take another example, efforts to compel institutions to provide services to categories or classes of clients for whom services are disproportionately costly is unlikely to succeed unless the regulatory body offers some rewards in exchange.

Writing service requirements into institutional charters, or establishing fines for noncompliance with legislative mandates to provide service, will not improve the effectiveness of regulation in that regard, and will not alone be sufficient to meet policy goals. Such actions are, in other words, inherently limited devices.

The technique of multiple, simultaneous comparisons can also reveal the limits of existing policies. As has been suggested several times, a system of vendor payments creates massive resource transfers from the public to the private sector with only the most minimal regulatory content—which almost invariably degenerates.

A Quick Look at Some Problems of Federalism

In many respects, grants-in-aid programs fit the model of regulation through contracting, with the signal exception that the regulatees are constitutionally sovereign states, rather than private firms or individuals. For historical reasons, much of the federal involvement in the delivery of health services has been effected through grants-in-aid programs, with the usual disadvantages of contracting (likelihood of inadequate enforcement, high costs, limitations of sanctions) magnified by the political status of the grantees.

It is fair to say that attempts at stringent regulation through intergovernmental grants-in-aid are inimical to healthy federalism. The creation of adversary relationships and a climate of mutual distrust is the only alternative to hypocritical nonfeasance by those charged with regulatory powers. That is not to say, however, that there is no role for the states in the regulation of the health sector, only that intergovernmental grants-in-aid are the worst of both worlds. Because health-care markets are highly localized, much of the regulation that is specific to a given market might appropriately be lodged in the states. To the extent, for instance, that a utility-regulation model is deemed advisable, whether universally or in more limited number of jurisdictions, there seems to be general agreement that it is best administered by the individual states.[92]

Since the federal government will continue, however, to be the major purchaser of health care even within those localized markets, some federal regulatory role is unavoidable. Here the analysis of limits becomes useful, because it is clear that there is no contradiction between utility regulation at one level of the federal system and contracting at another. In other words, the federal government could well choose to enter into highly specified contracts with health facilities, and even groups of individual professionals, which are already subject to regulation by state authorities. Although conflicts would inevitably arise from the differing perspectives, the triparite (federal, state, and provider) bargaining likely to emerge would not necessarily be dysfunctional for anyone, as opposed to the kind of conflict that arises in vendor payment or grants-in-aid programs. Because contracting is an inherently more flexible device than law enforcement, and because the regulatees would be private institutions rather than sovereign states, conflict would remain manageable.

How to Control Health Costs

If *synoptic analysis* is defined as providing a "one best way" of designing public policy, the foregoing analysis obviously fails the test. No alternative, or set of alternatives, is likely to be entirely satisfactory; each has its attendant advantages and disadvantages. In at least one respect, however, the analysis presented here has not even been very incremental. It was argued at the very beginning that the primary source of the demand for regulation in the health sector was the problem of costs. Yet the elaboration and comparison of models of the regulatory process presented here suggests that *none* of the regulatory alternatives can do very much about the most basic issue.

Regulation can have a significant impact on allocational efficiency (generally negative), on the degree of equity in the distribution of benefits and rewards in the health-care system, on the level of quality of services, on the rate of technological change, and even on the quality of interpersonal relationships. But regulation cannot do very much about costs. Recognition of that fact may be the most useful product of comparative analysis of the kind performed here.

The comparisons suggest that there are powerful underlying imperatives—social, economic, and technological—at the root of the cost problem in modern health services. That is neither a very innovative proposition nor a very radical one. People now expect as a right a panoply of services many of which did not even exist several generations ago; the environmental and behavioral stresses of modern life create new morbidities as fast as health-care institutions learn to cope with the old ones; the decay of other caring institutions passes on more and more responsibility to a health sector ever less-equipped for that function. As economists are so fond of remind us, there is no free lunch.

That regulation cannot do very much about costs does not imply, however, that *nothing* can be done. Should there be a collective decision to set some limit, no matter where, on the amount of resources society is prepared to devote to health care, let the chips fall where they might, it could be done. Short of that, we will probably have to bump along with less than satisfactory halfway measures. As the analysis in preceding sections reveals, both utility regulation and contracting offer the possibility of *partial* solutions, with attendant disadvantages of some magnitude. The question is not whether the game should be played, but whether it is worth the candle. I believe the mess a combination of utility regulation and contracting would be likely to create is at least marginally more attractive than the mess we are now in.

Summary

The existing health-care system in the United States performs very poorly on the criterion of costs; questionably on efficiency, equity, and quality; and unambiguously well only in technological progressiveness. Experience from other sectors suggests that utility-regulation techniques would have only a marginal effect on prices and quality. They would be very effective at increasing the equitableness of resource distribution through cross-subsidization. The reliance of utility regulation on highly formalized quasi-judicial processes is probably socially disfunctional in the aggregate.

Regulation through licensing is already pervasive in the health sector, and its continued extension is unlikely to accelerate its contribution to high prices, inefficiency, and inequity. Proposals for the reform of licensing, or even its extension in the case of facilities, are unlikely to be of much benefit, however, with the exception that more rational licensing policies, combined with peer review, may have a positive impact on quality.

Law enforcement is a more limited technique, applicable only when precise standards are available. When such standards do exist, and when the conditions for the prevention of administrative degeneration prevail, it can be a highly useful tool, as in much so-called "health and safety" regulation. Its ability to control costs is, however, limited to that portion of cost that arises from dishonest or fraudulent behavior.

Contracting draws on the role of government as a monopsonist to effect regulatory goals. Although highly susceptible to corruption and degeneration, it can be quite effective as a means of attaining efficiency, equity, and quality objectives. Except for those circumstances in which competitive bidding is feasible, however, it is more likely to inflate costs than reduce them.

None of the available regulatory techniques can, in short, do very much about health-care costs. The only clear way to control total costs is probably to simply put a ceiling on them, either in the aggregate or through disaggregated price control. Nonetheless, the process of comparing alternative regulatory techniques is not without its uses. Trade-offs can be specified, nonobvious combinations suggested, disbenefits anticipated. Existing policies or policy alternatives, such as vendor payment systems, can be put into fuller perspective. If politics is the art of the possible, "multiple, simultaneous comparisons" can help to define the realm of possibility.

Part IV

Toward the Future: Politics and Possibilities

7

The Political Economy of National Health Insurance: Policy Analysis and Political Evaluation

M. Kenneth Bowler,
Robert T. Kudrle, and
Theodore R. Marmor

National Health Insurance and American Politics

First a campaign issue for Roosevelt on the Bull Moose ticket, universal national health insurance remains in 1976—64 years later—a controversial legislative issue.[1] The conflict over national health insurance (NHI), although substantively about medical-care financing, is best understood as an example of "redistributive" American politics. Such political conflict is characterized by the opposition of large national pressure groups with coalitions relatively stable over time. The disputes are markedly ideological in nature, with the political struggle centralized at the federal level and monitored by the national media. The disputes over Social Security, the long battle over federal aid to education, the fight over Medicare, and now the conflict about NHI, exemplify this type of political issue. The question of the scope of government involvement in organizing, financing, and redistributing social services is the fundamental theme in all of these seemingly disparate issues.

Conflict between the opposing coalitions of national interest groups over national health insurance has been both intense and emotional. For the major participants, it is the redistribution of income, influence, and status, along with the legitimacy of highly valued political beliefs and symbols that have been at stake in NHI debates. On one side are those whose basic objective has been to shift medical-care financing from privately controlled institutions to the federal government. A central theme in their argument has been that private financing of medical care has produced intolerable inequities in the distribution of medical services. From their perspective, universal government-financed health insurance is the most important missing element in the set of social-welfare programs initiated with the Social Security Act's social insurance and public assistance programs.[2] They have persistently argued that medical services should be prepaid through a national tax system ensuring everyone, regardless of socioeconomic circumstances, both equal access to needed care and freedom from fearfully expensive medical bills. This group includes a number of prominent individuals who for forty years have been advising Presidents and

Research support from the National Center for Health Services Research facilitated the revisions of this chapter.

members of Congress on social welfare matters and advocating government-financed health insurance.[a]

Historically, the large, industrial labor unions of the CIO, and later the United Auto Workers (UAW), have spearheaded the recurrent demands for NHI. More recently, their special aim has been to eliminate health-insurance costs, generally the most expensive fringe benefits, from contract negotiations with management. They are convinced that a compulsory, tax-financed health program would provide their membership with comprehensive coverage at lower cost to union families. The industrial unions and social-insurance reform leaders have been regularly bolstered by a loose coalition of liberal church, professional, service, and consumer organizations—intermittently united in their support of NHI.

Organizations representing physicians, hospitals, insurance companies, and other segments of the health industry have historically opposed comprehensive, government health insurance. They have regarded government-financed health insurance as a dire threat to their professional status and to the discretion they have traditionally had in providing and financing medical services. Anti-NHI groups have persistently argued that the market structure of American medicine is responsible for the high quality of care enjoyed by most Americans. Government-financed health insurance, they have alleged, means government-controlled, lower quality, more depersonalized medical service. Their major objective has been to prevent federal control over the financing of medical services. In that effort, the health-industry pressure groups have had allies from other conservative and business-oriented national organizations, ranging from the Chamber of Commerce and the National Association of Manufacturers to the Young Americans for Freedom. The continuing debate between these sides has thus raised familiar symbolic and ideological conflicts associated with the broad issue of the government's role in the private economy.

The historical NHI debate is thus extraordinary in its stability of interest-group alignment and argument. The current struggle over NHI is almost identical to that which took place in the debate over the Social Security Act of 1935, Federal Aid to Education, Medicare and Medicaid in 1964–65, and the Nixon welfare reform proposals (The Family Assistance Plan) in 1969–72. This strong commitment or opposition to NHI—and what it symbolizes in terms of legitimate government action—is as important as the economic interests in understanding the politics of national health insurance.

---

[a]This group includes Wilbur Cohen (Secretary of Health, Education, and Welfare, 1968–69), I.S. Falk (Social Security Administration, 1936–54), Robert Ball (Commissioner of the Social Security Administration, 1962–73), and Nelson Cruikshank (Advisory Council Social Security Financing, 1957–58/Health Insurance Benefits Advisory Council, 1965–72). This group includes those involved in the development of the Social Security Act of 1935 and almost every other social welfare program since then.

National health insurance, much discussed in political, academic, and public arenas, has rarely proceeded to the decision stage in the federal policy process. Discussion has generally not been carried out with the intention or expectation that the enactment of NHI legislation would immediately follow, but is done to relieve the pressure that interest groups have exerted on candidates, legislators, and Presidents to take a stand or begin legislative action on NHI. The debate at this stage is dominated by ideological charge and countercharge, by symbols and slogans portending a more hopeful or fearful future if the government's role in health care were expanded as advocated by the NHI reformers.[3] The key symbols have included assurances of greater equality and security under government-financed NHI versus threats of socialized medicine, government encroachment, reduced freedom of choice, lower quality medical care, and higher health costs. The purpose of all interested groups has been to get the attention and arouse the concern of leaders and the public and to engender an active, intense, emotional commitment to one side or the other in the NHI debate.[4]

The historically vitriolic debate over NHI has helped to maintain the bipolar coalition. The intensity of the struggle has been evident whenever legislative action seemed even remotely feasible. For two decades after World War II government health-insurance proposals—for all, the elderly, or the poor—were salient. The enactment of Medicare in 1965 brought a temporary halt to the long-standing cleavage between the coalitions, and for nearly five years the public discussion of medicine centered on the problems of implementing Medicare and Medicaid and dealing with the unprecedented level of inflation that followed their enactment. Nineteen hundred and sixty-eight was the first presidential election since World War II in which the candidates felt no compunction about ignoring whether or not they favored government initiatives in health insurance. That hiatus was temporary, but when the debate reemerged it was to be importantly shaped by the inflationary experience of the late 1960s.

National Health Insurance in the 1970s

The leading advocates of national health insurance in the early 1970s comprised the so-called Committee of 100, chaired initially by Walter Reuther of the United Automobile Worker's Union. These advocates renewed the pattern of treating national health insurance as the answer to the crisis in American medicine. Not only were some of the proponents and proposals familiar, but so were the ingredients of the debate. Medical-care problems were cited as if no dispute were possible. The sides polarized again on the right answers to the problems. Public choice, the nation was told, consisted in selecting the proper response to the crises in cost, distribution, access, and quality of American medical care. The debate was structured as if the solutions were reasonable responses to worsening conditions; in fact, the reverse was true. Proponents of national health-insurance plans employed descriptions of crises to justify proposals whose central eligibility, administrative, and financing provisions were framed out of long-standing political and ideological conviction.

The Rhetoric of Crisis

Claims of a crisis in American medicine have intensifed in the last half decade. Specters of breakdown have accompanied nearly all of the recent NHI proposals. Although an effective and often used technique in mobilizing public opinion, the appeal to crisis impedes the appraisal of competing policy measures and their anticipated effects. The current debate over national health insurance has been no exception to this pattern.

The crisis rhetoric is bipartisan. The Republican administration, referring to the American medical-care system in 1969, warned that "unless action is taken, both administratively and legislatively . . . within the next two to three years, we will have a breakdown in our medical care system with consequences affecting millions of people throughout this country."[5] Senator Edward Kennedy's book *In Critical Condition* captured the views of many politicians about the problems of American patients in the 1970s. In a series of articles on "Our Ailing Medical System," *Fortune* magazine alleged that "American medicine, the pride of the nation for many years, stands . . . on the brink of chaos."[6] Labor leaders have maintained almost ritualistically that "there is little [they] can add in the way of new facts and figures to further prove what is generally accepted: that there is a medical care crisis in America."[7]

Opinion surveys in the early 1970s suggested that a large majority of Americans agreed there was a health crisis but did not regard it as their own. But they have worries: access to a physician, waiting time, cost, and impersonality.[b] Other polls indicate concern—particularly among physicians—about catastrophic financial consequences of serious or lingering illness, understandable since a large proportion of the population—under work-related or Medicare insurance—do not have adequate major medical protection.[8]

---

[b]Ronald Andersen et al., "The Public's View of the Crisis in Medical Care: An Impetus for Changing Delivery Systems?" *Economic and Business Bulletin* 24 (Fall 1971), pp. 44–52. See also Aaron Wildavsky, "Doing Better and Feeling Worse," Working Paper No. 19, Graduate School of Public Policy, University of California, Berkeley, March 1975, p. 2. The intensity of the health-care issue is increasing. Between 1972 and 1975 the proportion of those who regarded health care as a critical problem increased from 42 to 55 percent. Fifty-five percent of the respondents ranked health care as a "very, very important" issue (5 on a 5 point scale) compared with 42 percent three years ago. See remarks by Dorothy Lynch in National Health Council, *A Declaration of Interdependence: Developing America's Health Policy*, Proceedings of the Twenty-Fourth Annual National Health Forum, March 16–17, 1976, Philadelphia, Pennsylvania, p. 36.

Nevertheless, it is not patient concern about access or catastrophe that dominates the crisis conception of American medicine before congressional committees. The problem highlighted there is one of overall cost, expressed in the testimony of government program managers, insurance-company executives, and union leaders. Hospitals and physicians are increasingly under attack as the alarm over rising medical-care costs leads to the question of how efficiently and effectively the health industry delivers its services.

Medical-Care Problems

This assertion of crisis and the listing of problems have become the standard prologue for national health-insurance advocates. National health insurance is required, they argue, because the cost, quality, and distribution of American medicine are so unsatisfactory.

There are serious problem areas, but even taken together it is unclear whether they constitute a generally worsening crisis. It is crucial to keep this clear when comparing the national health-insurance plans since they are justified as responses to the ostensible crisis. But the citation of these problems as if they were signals for a particular national health-insurance plan is misleading. The provisions of the plans, as discussed below, address different aspects of America's health concerns. What the NHI plans reveal is not agreement—on crisis, problem, or solution—but disagreement.

Cost. Consider, for example, the most frequently cited problem: rising medical-care costs. That total expenditures for medical care have increased explosively in the past two decades is undeniable. Americans spent more than $118 billion on medical care in fiscal year 1975.[9] That means average expenses per person of $558 in 1975, compared with $485 in 1974. The proportion of the Gross National Product (GNP) devoted to medical care increased by more than 80 percent in the past 20 years, from 4.6 percent to 8.3 percent in 1975.[10]

Cost treated as total national expenditure is the approach of statisticians not citizens. What Americans worry most about are the prices of particular items (the office visit, an appendectomy, the insurance premium) or the costs of a severe illness (cancer, a broken hip, cerebral palsy). They fear the consequences of medical inflation in these personal terms, linking rising prices with out-of-pocket costs to their own family. They worry about insurance benefits expiring just when it is essential—in the rare financially catastrophic cases.[c]

---

[c]Michael Meyer, *Catastrophic Illnesses and Catastrophic Health Insurance* (Washington, D.C.: The Heritage Foundation, Inc., 1974), p. 4. Fewer than 1 percent spend more than $5,000 a year on medical care.

Governments likewise are more concerned about their costs than total health expenditures. As table 7-1 illustrates, the public sector has become the largest source of payment for personal-health care. Governments at all levels now account for 40 percent and the federal government alone is approaching 30 percent of total health expenditures. The dramatic growth is particularly evident at the federal level. Ten years ago, Medicare and Medicaid represented federal budget outlays of $5.9 billion; in 1975, approximately $25 billion. Although the state and local share of personal-health expenditures stabilized around 12 percent between 1966 and 1974, the federal share doubled.[11]

Cost control preoccupies Medicare and Medicaid administrators, and other government departments rightly fear the impact of medical inflation on their nonhealth programs. Although government expenditures have increased, so have the needs of their poorer clientele. In fact, the real value of Medicaid benefits per capita—taking inflation into account—declined between 1968 and 1974 in spite of the annual dollar increases in program expenditures (table 7-2). So the "cost" problem as actually perceived is not one but three: costs to society, to individuals, and to government programs. With the major focus on costs, the financing provisions of national health-insurance plans have become the central issue in the debate among alternatives.

Along with, and largely because of, rapidly rising health costs and public-health expenditures there has been a significant increase in government efforts to regulate the health-care industry. A decade ago, the industry operated relatively free of federal regulation, with the exception of certain health and safety standards. Examples of recent regulatory actions by the federal government include the establishment of professional standards review organizations (PSROs), physician-dominated units charged with regulating the cost and quality of care provided under federally supported medical programs, and The Health Planning Act of 1975, which established a network of area-wide and state health-planning agencies empowered to review the appropriateness of existing institutional health services and guide the construction of new health facilities. Recently, the Department of Health, Education and Welfare issued final regulations under which Medicare reimbursement of physicians' fees is tied to a national economic index. Specifically, the regulations limit any increase in the amount recognized as the prevailing charge for a given physicians' service in a locality to an amount justified by the economic index.

In sum, a large number of people already depend upon publicly financed personal-health care as an increasing amount of the compensation received by health providers already comes from public rather than private sources. Approximately 42 cents of every health-care dollar spent in the country is now collected and distributed by public agencies, and nearly a quarter of the population—mainly those under Medicare and Medicaid—has some part of their personal-health needs financed out of public funds.[12] It is at least 10 years ago and $50 billion too late to prevent the intrusion of government into our private health-care system.

Table 7-1

The Growth of Personal Health-Care Expenditure by Source of Payment

(Dollar Sums in Millions)

| | | Private Sector | | | | | | Public Sector | | | |
| | | Out of Pocket | | Insurance Benefits | | Industry and Philanthropy | | State and Local | | Federal | |
Fiscal Year	Total	Amount	Percentage of Total	Amount	Percentage of Total	Amount	Percentage of Total	Amount	Percentage of Total	Amount	Percentage of Total
1950	$ 10,400	$ 7,107	68.3	$ 879	8.5	$ 312	3.0	$ 1,124	10.8	$ 979	9.4
1955	15,231	8,992	59.0	2,358	15.5	412	2.7	1,886	12.4	1,583	10.4
1960	22,729	12,576	55.3	4,698	20.7	525	2.3	2,828	12.4	2,102	9.2
1965	33,498	17,577	52.5	8,280	24.7	683	2.0	4,118	12.3	2,840	8.5
1966	36,216	18,668	51.5	8,936	24.7	720	2.0	4,542	12.5	3,349	9.2
1967	41,343	18,786	45.4	9,344	22.6	753	1.8	4,991	12.1	7,471	18.1
1968	46,521	19,098	41.1	10,444	22.5	780	1.7	5,797	12.5	10,401	22.4
1969	52,690	20,957	39.8	12,206	23.2	824	1.6	6,421	12.2	12,283	23.3
1970	60,113	24,272	40.4	14,406	24.0	890	1.5	7,142	11.9	13,403	22.3
1971	67,228	26,307	39.1	16,728	24.9	964	1.4	7,827	11.6	15,401	22.9
1972	74,828	28,141	37.6	18,620	24.9	1,035	1.4	8,906	11.9	18,126	24.2
1973	82,490	30,348	36.8	20,955	25.4	1,125	1.4	9,884	12.0	20,178	24.5
1974	90,088	31,310	34.8	24,100	26.8	1,220	1.4	10,499	11.6	22,959	25.5
1975	103,200	33,599	32.6	27,340	26.5	1,337	1.3	12,345	12.0	28,578	27.7

Source: Marjorie Smith Mueller and Robert M. Gibson, "National Health Expenditures, Fiscal Year 1975," *Social Security Bulletin*, February 1976.

Note: Amounts shown are smaller than total health-care expenditures due to exclusion of prepayment and administrative expenses and government public-health activities, which were approximately 15 percent of personal expenditures in 1975.

Table 7-2
Federal Outlays per Medicaid Recipient, Fiscal Years 1968–74
Total Outlays and Recipients in Thousands

	1968	1969	1970	1971	1972	1973	1974
Total outlays							
In current dollars	$1,805,883	$2,284,713	$2,726,845	$3,362,303	$4,426,444	$4,599,899	$5,827,064
In constant (1969) dollars	$1,922,642	$2,284,713	$2,539,438	$2,929,961	$3,650,583	$3,648,704	$4,404,845
Number of recipients of services	11,500	12,060	14,507	18,223	20,632	23,537	27,187
Outlay per recipient							
In current dollars	$157	$189	$188	$185	$215	$195	$214
In constant (1969) dollars	$167	$189	$175	$161	$177	$155	$162

Source: L.B. Russell et al., *Federal Health Spending: 1969-74* (Washington, D.C.: National Planning Association, 1974), table 54, p. 62; table 57, p. 64.

Maldistribution. American medical care is also attacked as disorganized, badly distributed, fragmented, losing patients "between the units." There are serious shortages of physicians in rural areas and the inner cities, and complaints about the decline of the traditional family doctor.[d] The ratio of doctors per 100,000 people in rural America is less than half that of the cities. Changes in medical-school training programs and the interests of medical-school students have encouraged those who advocate greater emphasis on primary care: that provided by general practitioners, internists, and pediatricians. For example, between 1968 and 1974, the number of first-year positions filled by primary-care training programs nearly doubled, from 4,600 to 8,800. In 1975, 56 percent of the 12,700 graduating medical students entered programs in primary-care fields.[13] These developments may, however, be less profound changes than they appear. The strong, long-term trend towards specialization has reappeared within the so-called primary-care fields, illustrated by the tendency of young internists to bypass general internal medicine in favor of subspecialties like hematology, oncology, and endocrinology. This trend is demonstrated by the sharp increase in the number of physicians taking subspecialty examinations by the American Board of Internal Medicine: 200 in 1970 to 2,000 in 1974.

Quality of Care. The quality of treatment usually comes to public attention through suits for malpractice and accounts of the high cost of malpractice insurance. But errors of medical competence may be rarer and cause less social harm than questionable and inefficient medical services. Drugs are not always prescribed wisely or in moderation; surgery is not always necessary. Experts are concerned that "so many [Americans] lose their appendices, their wombs, or their tonsils . . . without good cause."[14] All these malpractices and poor practices may divert time and money away from more cost-effective uses such as immunizations for children and prenatal checkups for mothers.

From criticism of questionable and inefficient practice it is but one short step to skepticism about all sophisticated medical care. This attitude reminds us of iatrogenic (physician-caused) disorders and places emphasis on environmental-reform, anti-smoking campaigns, and highway safety programs. From this standpoint national health insurance is not the appropriate focus; indeed, for some it is a "giant step sideways."[15] Some thoughtful authors worry that we will put scarce public resources into traditional and costly medical care at the very time that other ways to improve our health are available.[16]

---

[d]Only some 70,000 of the 295,000 practicing in the country are pediatricians or general practitioners. AMA, *Profiles of Medical Practice, 1974*, Reference edition (Chicago: American Medical Practice, 1974), pp. 95, 100.

All of these criticisms—many of which have merit—lend plausibility to the fear of breakdown. However, the litany of critical problems implies more agreement among public critics than, in fact, exists. The proposals for national health insurance reveal conflicting—not consensual—standards for assessing American medicine; the plans also represent genuine disputes about how to deal with the competing demands for greater access, improved quality, and less rapid increases in medical prices. Even if the problems were given similar weight, there would be little reason to predict that similar national health-insurance plans would be offered as solutions.

In fact, in spite of the rhetorical popularity of crisis language, there is no agreed-upon major problem in health care *except* high and apparently uncontrollably rising costs. The various other "problems" are just that—defects that any sensible analyst would recognize but not conditions uniformly worsening so as to justify a fear of disaster. This is particularly true about access, where the gap between rich and poor adults has been substantially reduced in the past decade (table 7-3). Appeals to an accepted crisis have supported hopes of rapid decision, which the prolonged political struggle over national health insurance has frustrated.

Competing NHI Remedies

The most straightforward way to describe national health-insurance proposals is to compare their benefits, beneficiaries, financing, and administrative arrangements along simple grids. HEW regularly publishes such digests of congressional proposals, and public finance experts attach cost estimates and impact projections to them. Although valuable and indeed necessary for appraising the particular features of various bills, such an approach skirts the political meaning of the strategic combinations that persistently recur.

Three basic types of bill now dominate the public debate over national health insurance. Reflecting fundamentally different ideological orientations, the bills can be usefully distinguished by the scope and degree of centralization of governmental authority over medicine they propose.

Minimal-Intervention Measures

The first group of proposals relies on minimum public control over the medical-care industry. All reflect the shared assumption among national health-insurance contestants that government should redistribute the current costs of illness. The American Medical Association (AMA) has prominently advocated plans of this sort. Its Medicredit proposal, first presented in the early 1970s

Table 7-3

Physician Visits Per Capita, by Age and Family-Income Group, Fiscal Years 1964, 1967, and Calendar Year 1969

Age and Income Group[a]	1964	1967	1969
All ages	4.5	4.3	4.3
Low income	4.3	4.3	4.6
Middle income	4.5	4.2	4.0
High income	5.1	4.6	4.3
Ratio, high income to low income	1.19	1.07	.93
Under 15 years			
Low income	2.7	2.8	2.8
Middle income	2.8	3.9	3.6
High income	4.5	4.4	4.3
Ratio, high income to low income	1.67	1.57	1.54
15 to 64 years			
Low income	4.4	4.6	4.8
Middle income	4.7	4.1	4.1
High income	4.9	4.6	4.2
Ratio, high income to low income	1.11	1.00	.88
65 Years and older			
Low income	6.3	5.8	6.1
Middle income	7.0	6.7	5.8
High income	7.3	6.5	7.5
Ratio, high income to low income	1.16	1.12	1.23

Source: Spyros Andreopoulos, ed., *Primary Care: Where Medicine Fails* (New York: John Wiley & Sons, 1974), p. 163.

[a]*Low income* is defined as under $4,000 in 1964 and under $5,000 in 1967 and 1969. *Middle income* is defined as $4,000 to $6,999 in 1964 and $5,000 to $9,999 in 1967 and 1969. *High income* is defined as $7,000 and above in 1964 and $10,000 and above in 1967 and 1969.

(table 7-4), was designed as a federal-tax subsidy of health-insurance premiums in hopes of stimulating the purchase of more comprehensive plans. It would have replaced the present tax deduction for medical-care expenses with a tax credit to offset in whole or in part the premiums of qualified health-insurance plans. The amount of the credit was graduated in reverse: the higher the income tax bracket, the lower the tax credit.

According to the Medicredit scheme, the American medical-care system would respond to a more broadly distributed capacity to buy its services. From that perspective the answer to financial inaccessibility of care was simply to increase consumer purchasing power, particularly among lower income groups. This approach was directed both at consumers without adequate health insurance

Table 7–4
AMA "MEDICREDIT" Plan (Fulton-Broyhill-Hartke Bill)

Program would provide credits against personal income taxes to offset the premium cost of a qualified private health-insurance policy providing specified benefits. Employers would be required to provide qualified policies to retain favorable tax treatment.

Benefits	Tax credits of 10 to 100 percent of the cost of qualified health-insurance policy; amount of credit depends on annual tax payments with higher benefits given to those with lower taxable income. Voucher certificates for purchase of insurance issued to those with little or no tax liability. Policies to provide 60 days hospitalization or (substituted on a 2 for 1 basis) skilled-nursing facility, physician care, dental care for children, home health services, laboratory and x-ray, ambulance service. Catastrophic coverage of unlimited hospital days and an additional 30 days in a skilled-nursing facility.
Population Covered	All U.S. residents on a voluntary basis.
Financing	Tax credits from federal general revenues. Employers must provide qualified policies to take full premium cost as a normal business deduction.
Cost Sharing	$50 deductible for hospital or skilled-nursing facility stay. 20 percent coinsurance for physician care, home health services, laboratory and x-ray, ambulance, dental care. For catastrophic coverage, a deductible that varies by income. Total coinsurance limited to $100 per family for combined physician-lab-x-ray services; $100 per family for hospital outpatient, home health, and ambulance; and $100 per family for dental care; Medicaid to pay all cost sharing for cash-assistance recipients.
Administration	Private carriers issue policies. State insurance departments certify carriers and qualified policies. HEW issues voucher certificates. New federal board establishes standards.

Sources: Saul Waldman, *National Health-Insurance Proposals: Provisions of Bills Introduced in the 93rd Congress July, 1974,* Department of Health, Education and Welfare, Publications No. (SSA) 75-11920, April 17, pp. 188–92.

and at providers worried about the stability of their financing. Its sanguine view of other medical-care problems left many critics preoccupied with Medicredit's omissions. Nevertheless, the plan itself would have astonished AMA critics a decade ago and generated complaints within the medical profession for its encouragement of more third-party medical financing.

Also within this class are proposals to provide insurance protection against financially catastrophic expenses. Other governmental programs and private-health insurance would cope with the rest of the medical-care industry's problems.[17] The catastrophic portion of the Long-Ribicoff bill covers hospitalization stays beyond 60 days and annual medical expenditures of more than $2,000 (table 7-5). The major-risk insurance proposal (MRI) by Martin Feldstein would protect against disaster while requiring direct patient payment for most medical

Table 7-5
Long-Ribicoff-Wagonner, Catastrophic Protection

A two-part program consisting of (1) a catastrophic-illness plan for the general population and (2) federal medical assistance for the poor and medically indigent.

	Catastrophic-Insurance Plan	*Medical-Assistance Plan*
Benefits	Hospital inpatient *after* first 60 days. 100 days of skilled-nursing facility care for persons who received catastrophic hospital benefits. Physician services, lab and x-ray, home health services. Medical supplies and ambulance services except Medicare limit of $250 per year for outpatient psychiatrists' services in a year retained.	Hospital inpatient care 60 days, skilled-nursing facility care, intermediate-care facility, physicians services, lab and x-ray, home health services. Full cost of benefits under catastrophic plan for recipients not covered by catastrophic insurance, and cost sharing for recipients who do have catastrophic insurance.
Population Covered	Persons insured or receiving benefits under social security.	Low-income individuals and families regardless of age or employment status, with aid to families who have incurred heavy medical expenses relative to income.
Financing	Special tax on wages and self-employment income subject to social security tax. Rate initially 0.3 percent to rise to 0.4 percent.	State and federal general revenues.
Cost Sharing	Coverage begins only when expenses reach specified catastrophic proportions (after first 60 days of hospitalization with unlimited further days covered and $21 per day copayment; skilled-nursing facility for those who have received catastrophic hospital benefits, with $10.50 per day co-payment). Total coinsurance limited to $1,000 annually per person; $2,000 medical deductible.	$3 copayment for first 10 visits to a physician per family.
Administration	Through the Medicare program with private carriers handling claims.	

Sources: Saul Waldman, *National Health Insurance Proposals,* pp. 22, 202–13; John Holahan, *Financing Health Care for the Poor* (Boston: D.C. Heath and Co., 1975).

expenses, thereby reducing the rate of medical inflation by inducing cost consciousness on the part of the patient and hence it is hoped by the doctor as well. Feldstein's MRI is a comprehensive, universal health-insurance policy with a very high deductible—it would pay only those medical bills that exceed 10 percent of income.[18] Quite similar to the Feldstein plan, although administered through the IRS as a tax-credit scheme for large medical expense, is the bill sponsored by Senator Brock of Tennessee.[19] Generally, the use of a deductible high in relation to average yearly medical expenditures seeks to combat medical inflation with consumer and physicial restraint. Yet even when the deductibles are income related they raise doubts about financial access for many national health-insurance advocates.

Major Government Action

In contrast to this first group of proposals are those that call for major intervention on the part of the federal government. The most ambitious is the Kennedy-Corman bill (table 7-6), which proposes a government monopoly of the health-insurance business. To ensure that "money would no longer be a consideration for a patient seeking any health service," the Kennedy-Corman plan would establish a national health-insurance program with universal eligibility and unusually broad coverage of service, financed jointly by payroll taxes and general revenues. There would be no cost-sharing by patients so that care under the plan would be "free" at the point of service with the federal government paying providers directly. Further provisions of the bill address problems of cost escalation (by limiting the total budget for medical care), distribution (by creating incentives for comprehensive health-service organizations and for health personnel in underserved areas), and quality (by policing the standard of care).[20]

Mixed Stragegies

The third and final group of proposals includes a mixture of strategies that call for increased government regulation and partial federal subsidy of the present medical-care system. The leading hybrid proposal to date is the Ford Administration's Comprehensive Health Insurance Plan (CHIP)

Table 7-6
Kennedy-Corman Bill

A universal health-insurance program administered by HEW, financed by federal general revenues and payroll taxes. Broad benefits with no cost sharing and few limitations. Would establish a national health budget under which funds would be allocated to regions and localities.

Population Covered	All U.S. residents, without regard to whether they have contributed to the program through taxes.
Benefits	Hospital care (limited for psychiatric inpatient care to 45 consecutive days per spell of illness), and 120 days of care in a skilled-nursing facility physicians (comprehensive including checkups, immunization, well-baby, and family-planning services; psychiatric is limited to 20 visits per spell of illness but unlimited if furnished by HMO, hospital OPD, or mental health clinic). Dentists for children under 15 and eventually for entire population. Home health services. Other health professionals. Laboratory and X-ray. Medical supplies and ambulance services. Optometrists and eyeglasses. Prescription drugs for chronic and other specified illness.
Financing	Tax on payroll (1.0%), unearned income (1.0%), self-employed (2.5%), with employers paying 3.5 percent tax. Income subject to tax is the first $15,000 per year for individuals, the total payroll for employers (state and local government do not pay employer tax). Federal revenues equal to the total receipts from taxes.
Cost Sharing	No deductibles or coinsurance.
Administration	Federal government, by a special board in HEW with regional and local offices to operate program.

Source: Waldman, *National Health Insurance Proposals,* pp. 14, 145–56; Holahan, *Financing Health Care for the Poor,* pp. 84–86.

(table 7-7). It combines efforts to expand insurance through mandating employer offerings, to rationalize Medicaid by requiring larger patient financial contributions as the incomes of welfare families rise, and to control costs by state regulation and the encouragement of prepaid group practices, now widely known as health maintenance organizations or HMOs.

The mandated employer plans are a way of insuring vast numbers of families for health expenses with a minimum impact on the federal budget. Employers under CHIP would, for example, be required to offer policies with broad benefits and to pay three-quarters of the premium. The employee would pay one-quarter

Table 7-7
CHIP-Ford Administration Plan

A three-part, voluntary program, which would include: (1) a plan requiring employees to provide private insurance for employees, (2) an assisted plan for low-income and high medical-risk families and individuals, (3) an improved federal Medicare program for the aged.

Benefits	Hospitalization; physician services; laboratory x-ray; prescription drugs and medical supplies; home health visits (100 per year); posthospital extended care (100 days per year); well child care to age 6; eye, ea, and dental care to age 13; family planning and maternity care; inpatient mental health, 30 full or 60 partial; outpatient mental health; 30 visits to community center; 15 to private practitioner.		
	Employee Plan	*Assisted Plan*	*Plan for Aged*
Population Covered	Full-time employees.	Low-income families, employed or unemployed. Families and employment groups who are high medical risks. All others who wish to enroll on payment of premiums.	Aged persons insured under social security.
Financing	Employer-employee premium (employer paying 75%).	Federal and state revenues, and premiums from enrollees according to family-income groups.	Payroll tax and premium payments by the aged (with federal and state financing of premiums for low-income aged).
Cost Sharing	Deductible of $150 per person, co-insurance 25 percent. Total cost sharing limited to $1,500 per year per family.	Maximum provisions as in employee plan but reduced according to individual or family income.	Deductible $100 per person, coinsurance 20 percent. Total cost sharing limited to $750 per person per year. Reduced cost sharing for lower income aged.
Administration	Insurance through private carriers supervised by states under federal regulations.	Administered states using private intermediaries, under federal regulations.	Administered by federal government.

Sources: T.R. Marmor, "The Comprehensive Health Insurance Plan of 1974," *Challenge*, December 1974; Waldman, *National Health Insurance Proposals*, pp. 4, 25–48; Holahan, *Financing Health Care for the Poor*, pp. 77–83.

of the premium and be responsible for substantial cost sharing at the time of use. More modest payment scales would obtain for families in lower income categories. Whatever the specific features, such plans share the current health expenditures among patients, employers, and the government; they do not lower health costs unless they result in less care (although they do lower government expenditures—a fact central to much of their political appeal). Furthermore, the increased attention to whether or not care is really needed in various circumstances, a supposed result of the considerable deductible, might be widely obviated through collective bargaining, as employers supplement the federally mandated plan.

Very similar to the administration's CHIP bill is the 1974 proposal of Senator Kennedy and Representative Wilbur Mills (table 7-8). Their scheme

Table 7-8
Kennedy-Mills Bill

A two-part program consisting of (1) a national health-insurance plan for the general population and (2) a revised Medicare plan for aged and disabled including a long-term care benefit.

	NHI	Medicare, Regular	Medicare, Long-Term
Benefits	Comprehensive, as in CHIP.	Comprehensive, as in CHIP.	Extensive provisions for home and institutional-care services.
Population covered	Persons insured or eligible for social security, working full-time or AFDC or SSI.	Aged and disabled, as under present Medicare program.	Aged and disabled, as under present Medicare program.
Financing	Payroll tax (3% for employers, 1% for employees) self-employment and unearned income (2½%) and AFDC and SSI payments. Income up to $20,000 taxable.	Continuation of same financing provisions.	Enrolled pay $6 monthly premium. Balance from federal and state revenues (90% and 10% respectively).
Cost sharing	Deductible $150 per person. Coinsurance $25. Total cost sharing limited to $1,000 per family but eliminated for low-income families. No cost sharing for preventive care.	Same as present Medicare program but eliminated or reduced for low-income families.	No cost sharing, except social security or SSI benefits reduced for persons receiving institutional services.
Administration	Administered by an independent SSA with insurance carriers processing claims.	Administered by an independent SSA with insurance carriers processing claims.	New community centers provide or arrange for services under state and SSA supervision.

Sources: Waldman, *National Health Insurance Proposals*, pp. 16, 161; Holahan, *Financing Health Care for the Poor*, pp. 86–90.

represented a more politically acceptable version of the Kennedy-Corman plan in the fiscally constrained bargaining of 1974. The Kennedy-Mills proposal is similar to CHIP in the structure of benefits and out-of-pocket payments. Where they differ most sharply is in their financing. The Kennedy-Mills program would be run by the Social Security Administration (as with Medicare), using the insurance industry as fiscal intermediaries. A 4 percent payroll tax (up to $20,000) would finance the program, with the employer nominally paying 3 percent and the employee not more than 1 percent. In addition, there would be a tax on self-employment and unearned income and on family-welfare payments, and miscellaneous state and federal contributions.[21] With such financing, the estimated *federal* cost of the Kennedy-Mills plan at $77 billion vastly exceeds that of the CHIP plan at $43 billion, although both are lower than the estimated $103 billion federal cost of the Kennedy-Corman plan (1974 estimates by the Secretary of HEW).

Another important difference is the impact by income classes of the two schemes. Most economists agree that much of compulsory premiums and payroll taxes are shifted to employees regardless of who nominally pays. Each employee under the administration plan gets charged an equal amount—the premium—but under the Kennedy-Mills plan the burden is in proportion to income, and explicit cost sharing is also more generous to the poor. The administration scheme thus takes much more from the relatively poor.[e] Like the administration plan, the Kennedy-Mills plan gives various financial incentives for the establishment of HMOs.

It is striking how the political debate over CHIP and the Kennedy-Mills plan—relatively close in substance—distorts their differences. The influence of ideology on the shape of the various bills makes comparison of proposals difficult. The proponents of all the various plans are apt to claim more for their bills than is possibly justified. National health insurance cannot solve all the shortcomings of the health industry. The problems are not only complicated, but solutions to one conflict with the solutions to another. One may not agree with AMA solutions, but the organization has recognized that improving "any system of medical care depends basically on balancing three strong and competing dynamics: the desire to make medical care available to all, the desire to control cost, and the desire for high quality care."[22] The competition among these goals is such that serving any two of them works against the third:

when you link the quest for ready and universal access with a desire to maintain quality of care . . . that combination of factors works against cost controls . . . If

---

[e]Although some of the tax falls on the wage earner, some appears to be shifted forward resulting in the raising of goods prices. Hence, a part of the tax becomes a kind of consumption tax spread around the community. For an estimate of the relative incidence of the administration scheme in comparison with Kennedy-Mills, based on the assumption of complete shifting to the wage earner, see Karen Davis, *National Health Insurance* (Washington: The Brookings Institution, 1975, pp. 147-150).

you link quality with vigorous efforts to control costs, then there has to be pressure on access. . . . [23]

Values and Causality in the Analysis of National Health-Insurance Alternatives: An Illustration

In spite of the ideological wrangling, there is good reason to believe that more than "half-truth" advertising messages of competing interest groups make the discussion of national health insurance a difficult one for informed public debate. In 1971 Martin Feldstein presented his analysis of America's medical problems in an article in the *Public Interest;* in February 1975 *Consumer Reports* evaluated the direction the nation should take on health insurance.[24] These two discussions are worth our careful attention for two reasons. First, among those presentations not launched directly from Congress or the executive branch, they will probably be among the most influential evaluations of our present situation and measures to improve it. Second, the two pieces present a dramatic contrast in thinking about medical care, and the assumptions of both, implicit as well as explicit, typify two opposing mindsets with which those following the health-insurance debate will become increasingly familiar. Although Feldstein presents his own solution, Consumers' Union opts for one of the two Kennedy proposals (Kennedy-Corman or Kennedy-Mills).

As noted earlier the plan proposed by Feldstein consists of major risk insurance (MRI) which in its simplest formulation would pay for all of a very broad range of medical expenditures once a certain out-of-pocket expense limit was reached. Reimbursement would be to consumers, and the expenditure limit would be geared to family income with perhaps 10 percent of annual income at risk (up to a certain fixed maximum). The problem of having enough cash on hand to cover expenditures below the limit would be dealt with by the ability of the individual or family to use government-guaranteed credit. A variant of the plan Feldstein favors is to have a lower deductible, perhaps 5 percent of family income, followed by 50 percent coinsurance over another 10 percent of income. The advantage of this more complex scheme is to keep persons partly financially responsible even for high medical expenditures; the rationale for this will become apparent below. The scheme could be administered by present insurance carriers.

Both discussions present well-defined sets of goals for future public policy towards health insurance reproduced in table 7-9, and much can be learned by focusing our discussion on them. The first two goals of both sets relate to how the medical system should confront the consumer in need of care, and the discussions of the two points cover some of the same ground. Both reject piecemeal reform schemes (such as the present administration's plan), which they allege could provide different kinds of medicine for the rich and the poor.

Table 7-9
Essential Health-Insurance Features

Feldstein	Consumer's Union
An acceptable plan should:	
1. Prevent deprivation of care because of inability to pay	1. Everyone's health-care needs should be covered, and the entire population should be included (universal, mandatory and unitary).
2. Prevent financial hardship	2. There should be no connection between a patient's income and the extent or quality of care dispensed.
3. Keep costs down	3. The plan should be financed progressively and in a manner open to public scrutiny.
4. Avoid a large tax increase	4. The program should provide incentives for efficiency, control over cost and quality, and encourage innovation.
5. Be easily administered	5. Administrators should be accountable to the public and consumers should have a voice in administration.
6. Be generally acceptable	

Sources: Martin Feldstein, "A New Approach to National Health Insurance," *The Public Interest,* Spring 1971; "National Health Insurance: Which Way to Go?" *Consumer Reports,* February 1975.

Both recognize the present problems of inadequate insurance for the middle class (and the failure of the administration's plans in this regard, particularly with respect to between-job coverage). Both discussions consider cost-sharing arrangements—although the difference in approach is striking.

Although Feldstein sees cost sharing as the most important single instrument for improving the entire system, CU regards the practice with much suspicion. CU is concerned over whether or not cost-sharing would serve most effectively to reduce *initial* demand by those needing medical attention or to increase cost consciousness in the delivery of medical services. Feldstein's discussion does not even consider the former possibility, but CU argues that, if initially tried, there should be no cost sharing for the poor or for preventive care for everyone. Furthermore, CU holds that out-of-pocket payments should be jettisoned immediately if they can be shown "to deter persons from seeking needed care."

The different attitudes towards cost sharing are shown to be based on a fundamental difference in approach, which we argue represents perhaps the major watershed in the discussion of national health insurance, and it partly evident in the very different treatments the two discussions give to the issue of cost levels for health care. Both Feldstein and CU are concerned with the level and the rate of change of costs in the medical sector, but their analyses could scarcely be more different. In Feldstein's view (based in large part on his own econometric research), the greatest single cost issue is that consumers and doctors have insufficient interest in controlling costs at the time of treatment because payment is made by third parties. The growth of private and government insurance has been the principal cause of inflation in the past, and, if present trends continue—ones that plans such as that of the AMA would accelerate—the situation can only get worse. Feldstein's answer is essentially to reverse the type of coverage provided by the present insurance system. Instead of immediate and inclusive insurance (for hospitalization particularly), which may nonetheless run out, what is needed is a system that keeps the average consumer paying a large part of *average*, annual health-care expenditure (only a few hundred dollars a year) but protects against large bills.

Furthermore, Feldstein is concerned about the impact of increased taxes, fearing that national income may be lowered. CU warns that "most cost estimates are unreliably partisan" and implies that the only important issue is "new spending for medical care." In doing this CU is technically in error and could be accused of misleading its readers—additional costs do result from giving things away "free" and paying for them with tax revenue. Just as a tax on cigarettes changes their price relative to other things and presumably how many of them are purchased, so, too, does an increase in the tax upon work— either a payroll or an income tax—change the terms upon which work is traded off for leisure. Nevertheless, the distortion of the supply of work effort engendered by the taxes necessary to finance the very substantial difference in federal expense between Feldstein's proposed major-risk insurance, perhaps $10 billion, and the much higher federal price tag of a scheme like Kennedy-Griffiths or Kennedy-Mills is not clear.[f] CU—and the public—might thus be forgiven for being more concerned about other issues—concerning power and choice mechanisms—connected with running health-insurance monies through the federal budget than with its distortion of work-leisure choices.

CU's third criterion really involves two different considerations. On the issue of progressive financing, the Feldstein plan financed through general federal

---

[f]Experts in public finance differ not only in their assessment of the magnitude of changed behavior resulting from increases in taxes but even the direction. When the tax on cigarettes goes up, most people buy fewer of them—the only question is how many fewer. When taxes lower the net hourly earnings of a person, however, the impact is not predictable solely on the basis of theory. On the one hand, the price of giving up an hour of work to take an hour of leisure has gone down, but it is also possible that the newly impoverished person may now have less enthusiasm for leisure relative to other goods and services. This is not the end of the complication, however. The use of the monies determines which parts of society—if any—actually feel poorer than before the tax hike was instituted. Whatever happens, the choices of individuals are still distorted by the income tax, as they are by virtually all taxes.

revenues with a proportional deductible and coinsurance would come off well, and the Kennedy-Corman bill gets high marks. The Kennedy-Mills plan and particularly the administration plan do less well. The openness to public scrutiny standard appears to be aimed mainly at the AMA plan with its reliance on largely unsupervised tax credits.

CU's fourth concern, incentives for efficiency, innovation, and quality is presented in a way that contrasts sharply with the Feldstein approach. Feldstein's basic position implies that medicine is an industry dominated by a "technostructure"—the persons who call the shots are fascinated by technological innovation and involve themselves in it as much as possible.[g] Consumers rely heavily on the advice of the doctor and, with an almost completely insured patient, the doctor pursues the "highest quality" of medical care without concern about visiting a financial hardship on his subject. Feldstein holds that, for most of the patient population, the increased sophistication of facilities and treatment have contributed relatively little to increased well-being, and much of it would never have been supplied if the patient were responsible for a larger part of the payment for a typical episode of treatment. Furthermore, cost-conscious patients and doctors would move increasingly towards new modes of organization such as health-maintenance organizations (presuming they offer genuine economies in delivery) if, as Feldstein recommends, the actuarial value of the major-risk insurance policy could be applied to the annual HMO charge.

CU's skepticism about cost sharing is reflected in its attention to other mechanisms to control costs. It recommends direct controls including negotiated budgets for institutions and negotiated fee schedules for practitioners—unfortunately little is said about the exact criteria by which these schedules should be determined. There would be explicit incentives for the introduction of organizational innovations like HMOs, and peer review of medical practice appears to be endorsed.

The statement of criterion 5 in each list appears to have resulted from the form of the final proposed plan. The CU plan is not simple or cheap to administer (which CU openly admits and laments) and therefore the best that can be hoped for is high accountability; the Feldstein plan is cheap both because there is virtually no administrative discretion and because only a minor fraction of total medical-payment transactions would need to be handled through third parties.

---

[g]The term, of course, is that of John Kenneth Galbraith in his *New Industrial State* (Boston: Houghton Mifflin, 1967). Few economists were persuaded of the substantial area of autonomy for most of the industrial sector, which characterizes Galbraith's presentation. It appears never to have been pointed out, however, that medicine may be the one major industry in which the "revised sequence"—the virtual determination of demand by producers—is more than a myth.

Feldstein's point 6, general acceptability, reflects mainly the fact that the perceived threat to the medical community is lower in his scheme than in nearly all others except that proposed by the AMA. This criterion is open to question, however, in that although most medical practitioners are not keen on the Kennedy proposals, it is not at all clear that their misgivings would undermine the plans.

It was suggested earlier that the two discussions differ profoundly in their basic approach, and the difference turns upon the nature of medical care itself. Rashi Fein has observed that "health is different."[25] Virtually every major group and analyst is willing to admit that health care is not just another product, and this recognition is as old as the Hippocratic oath. Having admitted the special character of medical care, however, analysts appear to take two very different approaches to it. For Feldstein, health care is different mainly because it is *fundamental*. Indeed, he explicitly justifies public attention to it because of its similarity to food and shelter. The approach taken by Consumers Union and virtually all "liberal" observers goes a critical step further. Health care, is, of course, fundamental but in addition it is for the typical consumer intrinsically *incomprehensible:* the nature of need and of proper treatment is so beyond the power of the consumer adequately to evaluate so as to set it in a category apart from food and shelter.

The acceptance or rejection of the notion of the informed rational consumer is difficult to overestimate in contrasting the two positions. It is Feldstein's trust in the consumer's informed rationality that lies at the basis of his entire analysis. When proper incentives are present, the doctor functions as something of a personal "brain trust" on health—one who can provide a meaningful discussion of alternatives to which the consumer can sensible respond. The increased "early" dollar payment is not meant solely to make the doctor careful out of a sense of responsibility for his patient but also because of the increased shopping around in which the consumer is expected to engage. If his fee is too high or the advice he gives too expensive, another such consultant can be found. To the extent that the patient does this little or not at all the restraint on soaring costs will be weakened. For CU the notion of rational consumer choice in medicine must be largely an illusion. Remembering that CU rejects cost-sharing for the poor and insists on free preventive medicine (the latter is also considered by Feldstein), how otherwise can one explain CU's fear that coinsurance might "deter persons from seeking needed care?" The only conclusion is that if the consumer faces the real cost of alternatives, he may very well make the *wrong* choice—to call it wrong indicates that the consumer's judgment is not to be trusted.

Another element of irrationality (actually extreme risk aversion) could vitiate the entire system. Feldstein assumes that the several hundred dollar difference for a typical consumer between the expected payment in any one year and the maximum payment under his scheme will not result in the purchase of additional insurance by a typical consumer. If it does not, there will be self-selection of the additional coverage by those families with a high expected expenditure and the premium will rise, thus further discouraging insurance by most potential purchasers. Unfortunately, as Feldstein admits, it is possible that a very large percentage of people will buy the additional insurance, in spite of his proposed elmination of all tax advantages for such purchase. If they do the entire scheme loses most of its rationale.

It may appear that there is a clear-cut difference in the extent of consumer rationality assumed—or sovereignty accepted—and that the policy implication for those who reject it is zero-price medicine. The issue is not quite so simple. Assume, as Feldstein undoubtedly does, that the number of people who would be deterred from seeking needed medical aid (as determined by some polling of consumers and doctors) would not be strictly zero. What is often suggested as a conclusive solution—and this is implicit in the CU analysis—is that the problem would be remedied with a zero charge. A moment's reflection, however, suggests it is in fact very unlikely that the zero charge is sufficiently "low" to induce the "correct" behavior. Many persons would still not make the social and in some cases economic sacrifices necessary for appropriate medical attention (all of the costs of being "out of commission" for a period) even at a zero price. Only a substantial subsidy would suffice, and most would grant that this is presently a political impossibility.

The perhaps seemingly fatuous point just made actually suggests another important divergence in thinking about medical care. Many writers with attitudes similar to those evidenced in the CU discussion place little stress on the fact that medical care is only a minor part of the total health picture and that, as was hinted earlier, a strong case can be made that many public and private actions (involving, for example, safety regulations or dietary habits) might be more cost-effective in creating better health than a medical-care system with zero prices— even assuming the actual volume of medical attention for a typical patient is increased in response to increased demand. This last assumption is dubious at best. If direct purchasing power is removed from the medical market, it is quite possible that a lower volume of medical resources might ultimately result from the governmental payment for, and political decisions about, their provision. The recent underfunding of the British National Health Service illustrates the problem.

Competing Problems and Competing Remedies

The preceding discussion stressed the issue of consumer payment to illustrate fundamentally different approaches to our present problems. Let us return now to our original concerns about cost distribution and quality of care and use them to examine the health-insurance proposals being actively considered.

Cost

What will any of the proposals do about the rate of inflation in medical care prices and continuing increases above our current health expenditures of over $100 billion per year? Should we not be spending more on medicine, as we get richer? Moreover, it may well be that medical care is what economists call an "elastic" good, meaning that, holding prices and technical conditions constant, people will spend *relatively* more on medical care as their per-capita income goes up. Therefore (if those conditions held) increases in relative expenditures would occur over time under any system that really reflected the preferences of its citizens. Another consideration is that, as a society becomes richer, the purchase of time of a typical citizen in his role as producer must go up—that, after all, is what increasing per-capita income means. To the extent that unit prices of outputs in the medical sector reflect labor time, they must go up. Additionally, an unknown amount of the increase in the unit price of medical-care services we have experienced doubtless represents an increase in quality.

Although many accept that these factors in combination would yield rising relative expenditures over time even if consumers incurred charges as they do in other markets, it is a widely held suspicion—clearly expressed in the Feldstein analysis of rising costs—that medical-care practitioners are presently "administering" a more expensive level of care than would ever be chosen by most patients if they faced the bill at the time of choice rather than earlier when they paid their insurance premiums. The AMA approach of yet more conventional insurance alarms a broad spectrum of opinion, and even those who reject the kind of consumer preference Feldstein's approach typifies usually express the view that there are unnecessary frills or excessive salaries that inflate medical bills.

Although some, including Senator Kennedy, stress that we can clamp down on medical inflation *only* through *complete* federal financing, the experience in Canada and Sweden suggests that merely having governments finance the bulk of medical-care services will not in itself reverse the prevailing upward spiral in prices and expenditures.[h] There is evidence, however, that when financing is concentrated at one governmental level *and* service providers are directly budgeted (rather than reimbursed by insurance), expenditures and their rate

---

[h]See Odin Anderson, *Health Care: Can There Be Equity?* (New York: John Wiley & Sons, 1973), for evidence on postwar price and expenditure trends in England, Sweden, and the United States. A recently published work, *National Health Insurance: Can We Learn From Canada?* Spyros Andreopoulos, ed. (New York: John Wiley & Sons, 1975), documents the financing role of public authorities in Canada and their frustration over the past decade in curbing expenditure and price increases to anything below that of the United States. See particularly chapter 3 by R.G. Evans. See also T.R. Marmor, D.A. Wittman, and T.C. Heagy, "Politics, Public Policy, and Medical Inflation," in Michael Zubkoff, ed. *Health: A Victim or Cause of Inflation,* (NY: Milbank Memorial Fund, 1975).

of increase are lower. With its National Health Service, England has spent in the last 15 years a third less of its resources on medical care and experiences roughly a third the expenditure increases relative to the GNP of Canada, Sweden, or the United States (table 7-10).[1] To the 16 percent of Americans who favor putting doctors on salary in an English-style system, this will be a welcome argument.[26] But even to others, the experience of Great Britain suggests a financing concentration desirable in a future national health-insurance program. Thus, the "conservative" emphasis on controlling inflation may best be accomplished by a greater degree of governmental centralization than even many "liberals" favor.

Of the leading United States plans, the Kennedy-Corman bill—with its concentrated[j] federal financing—affords the best theoretical prospects for

Table 7-10
Total Expenditures for Health Services as a Percentage of the Gross National Product, Seven Countries, Selected Periods, 1961-73

Country	WHO Estimates[a]		SSA Estimates[b]		McKinsey Estimates[c]	
	Year	Percentage of GNP	Year	Percentage of GNP	Year	Percentage of GNP
Canada	1961	6.0	1969	7.3	1970–73	7.7
United States	1961–62	5.8	1969	6.8	1970–73	7.7
Sweden	1962	5.4	1969	6.7	1970–73	7.0
Netherlands	1963	4.8	1969	5.9	1970–73	7.3
Federal Republic of Germany	1961	4.5	1969	5.7	1970–73	6.1
France	1963	4.4	1969	5.7	1970–73	5.8
United Kingdom	1961–62	4.2	1969	4.8	1970–73	5.3

[a]Brian Abel-Smith, *An International Study of Health Expenditure,* WHO Public Paper No. 32, (Geneva: 1967.

[b]Joseph G. Simanis, "Medical Care Expenditures in Seven Countries," *Social Security Bulletin* (March 1973), p. 39.

[c]Robert Maxwell, *Health Care: The Growing Dilemma,* 2nd ed. (New York: McKinsey and Company, June 1975), pp. 18, 68.

---

[i]See T. Marmor, T. Heagy, and W. Hoffman, "National Health Insurance: Some Lessons from the Canadian Experience," *Policy Sciences,* special issue on comparative policy research, 6, no. 4 (December 1975), pp. 447–466. This article is a revised version of the one by Marmor in Andreopolous, *National Health Insurance: Can We Learn from Canada?* chapter 4. More specifically on inflation controls, see Marmor, Wittman, and Heagg, "Politics, Public Policy, and Medical Inflation."

[j]By concentration we mean a single unit of government paying the bill—the Health Security Board in the case of the Kennedy-Corman bill. By contrast, our present medical financing is dispersed among patients, numerous insurance carriers, and federal, state, and local government agencies.

curbing inflation. But to be effective, it must be fully implemented, which is at present unlikely. The Feldstein plan is directed at cost containment placing financial responsibility on patients to restrain inflation. But to work, such a plan must discourage supplementary insurance—a daunting political task.[k] Hence, the most promising anti-inflation proposals are politically the least likely to emerge in the United States. More likely is CHIP or some other mixed plan, which would offer more business and further subsidies to health-care insurers and providers without strict central budgetary control. This fiscally decentralized plan would be inflationary yet would still leave major gaps in coverage: the worst of both worlds. Thus it appears that the national health-insurance scheme initially adopted in the coming years will offer little hope for controlling costs: a real market solution *or* effective bureaucratic controls each in its own way appears too "radical" to emerge from the pulling and hauling of impending congressional deliberation.

Maldistribution

National Health insurance is likely to be more successful in improving access than in containing costs. But financial barriers are only part of the problem. Equally serious is unavailability of care in major areas and specialties, the result of poor distribution of medical personnel.[27] No proposed remedy has worked well—neither educational loan forgiveness for service in underdoctored areas, nor substitution of rural or ghetto medical service for physicians' military obligations, nor subsidies for medical centers in underserved locales. Other Western democracies have learned that poor distribution remains after the medical purchasing power of poor city neighborhoods and remote rural areas are improved.[28] Only Draconian-forced assignment to regions and specialties would work;[l] otherwise young doctors have good professional and social reasons for continuing to prefer specialty practices in affluent suburban neighborhoods.

Many observers have claimed that with the current supply of doctors, at least in primary care, there is chronic excess demand,[29] thus giving doctors much discretion in their behavior. The usual "doctor-shortage" analysis is that doctors do not ration by price as much as they do so by exercising wide choice in location—thus increasing queues in some places and reducing them in others—and by picking and choosing interesting or challenging, rather than routine,

---

[k]Interviews with HEW officials suggest that any effort to *change* the current tax advantages of health insurance meet with fierce resistance. This resistance has led Stuart Altman, deputy assistant secretary for health, Office of Planning and Evaluation, HEW, to conclude that more drastic constraints on insurance would have a near-zero probability of enactment.

[l]No absolute minimum ratio of doctors to patients has ever been agreed upon, and the notion of geographic equality—at whatever the national average—is not sensible because there will always be heavy concentrations of personnel at regional medical centers.

work. More rationing by price may be retarded by the doctor's sense of responsibility towards his patient. Many have argued, however, that a doctor's influence over his patients' "needs" makes expanding physician supply a chancy and expensive corrective strategy. Thus, one school says that a way of avoiding skyrocketing costs with national health insurance is to increase physician supply and the other argues that each new doctor will be able to "earn" the going rate and thus add to costs! There is no conclusive evidence on the issue one way or the other, and we are confronted with an area of vital importance to national health insurance in which expert opinion points us in opposite directions. Thus, it is perhaps not surprising that none of the national health-insurance proposals addresses the personnel question very forcefully.

A further complication is that the efficacy of the increased supply solution in dampening costs is not independent of the insurance scheme proposed. The more conventional economic solution is more persuasive where the doctor and the patient are both maximally concerned about costs. In other words, the solution of increasing supply appears most plausible under a scheme such as that of Feldstein and least promising under a plan like that of the AMA. HMOs also appear to offer hope that increased supplies of personnel would put downward pressure on prices (and would produce other improvements as well), but our assessment here founders on our inability to forecast with certainty just how HMOs will actually prosper under the various plans that encourage their formation.

Quality of Care

National health insurance, whether fiscally centralized or decentralized, is unlikely to transform the quality of medical care. It may provide incentives for preventive care,[m] but it cannot check malpractice or doubtful practice much better than present institutions do. Moreover, the enforcement of minimum "quality" standards may actually stimulate the demand for costly and inefficient procedures. The quality of medical care depends much more on professional

---

[m]It should be noted that there is little evidence to support the general enthusiasm for preventive care. There are indications that primary prevention—for example, prenatal care—effectively prevents some maternal, infant, and child problems. But there is evidence that mass screening programs and even the annual physical checkups are economically wasteful and only occasionally detect conditions that are aided by early treatment. Economists Burton Weisbrod and Ralph Andreano conclude that preventive care can increase costs without significantly raising the level of health. Apparent cost savings in the Kaiser-Permanente plan (which is often cited as a model of the medical and financial efficacy of prevention) they attribute to "various factors, many of which are unrelated to preventive care." Ralph Andreano and Burton Weisbrod, *American Health Policy: Perspectives and Choices* (Chicago: Rand McNally, 1974), p. 35.

self-regulation and consumer awareness than on any conceivable health-insurance plan's regulations. Adequate financing cannot ensure that the care received is good.

This skepticism about national health insurance's capacity to reform American medical care need not justify public-policy inaction. The major aim of insurance is to calm fears of financial disaster. Other issues are peripheral to that concern. The argument that more traditional medical care will not markedly improve our health is beside the point when one asks whether the current burden of medical-care expenses is sensibly distributed. Some have argued that national health insurance without incentives for prevention and improvement of health is not worth having. But would anyone seriously argue that automobile insurance, for example, is not worth having if it does not prevent accidents and improve the quality of our automobiles?

Recognizing the conflicting objectives in national health-insurance proposals is the prerequisite for a rational debate over NHI. The choices include whether the United States should spend a larger share of its resources on medical-care services, through the federal government or otherwise. Should efforts be made to make care more accessible (and perhaps less fancy), or substantially higher quality (and, therefore, more expensive), and should the use of medical care be independent of ability to pay (and, therefore, likely to be more costly in the aggregate)?

The debate over national health insurance will be a particularly obscure and frustrating one for all Americans interested in health insurance mainly as consumers and taxpayers. First, most of the political rhetoric tends to concentrate on the symbols rather than on the substance of the alternative proposals. This is nowhere more evident than in the administration's strong opposition to the Kennedy-Mills proposal when in fact its own plan is very similar, except that the Democratic proposal runs the necessary funds through the federal budget and the other calls for the purchase of private insurance. Further, a close look at the proposals reveals important differences of both values and assumed causality. If only the former were at issue, a large number of persons could probably take sides with confidence, but the empirical matters involved are so murky that most careful observers will probably have their diligent attention to the subject rewarded, not with understanding, but with higher levels of confusion. Finally, there are important issues in the medical-care area about which much ink has been spilled to which none of the proposed health-insurance plans offers any real hope of solution.

Changing Legislative Politics and the Prospects for National Health Insurance

During the early 1970s Congress dealt only sporadically with national health insurance. The House Ways and Means Committee began an important set of hearings on NHI in April 1974; this was the first formal legislative action on the subject since 1971. After several months of intermittent hearings, Wilbur Mills, chairman of the Ways and Means Committee, announced that the committee would begin making decisions and drafting NHI legislation on August 5. After several days of staff briefings and general discussion, the committee members were presented with a "compromise" NHI proposal that had been drafted at Mills' instructions by the staff of the committee and the Department of Health, Education and Welfare.

This proposal was an effort by Mills to produce a consensus within the committee. It included features of many of the major NHI bills and a number of provisions that had been advocated by different members of the committee during the hearings and committee discussion. On the basic issue of financing, it attempted to split the difference or provide a compromise by combining the Long-Ribicoff, federal catastrophic-health program with the mandated, private-insurance coverage contained in the Nixon administration's NHI bill. This would have established a federally financed and administered catastrophic health-insurance plan requiring employers to provide their workers a standard package of *private* health-insurance protection covering basic or noncatastrophic health needs. The required private-insurance coverage would be underwritten and operated by insurance companies, and employers would pay 75 percent of the insurance premium. Because it would expand both public and private financing of health care, it was hoped that the proposals might provide the basis for a compromise on the key issue of financing.

As one might expect from the foregoing analysis, the major interest groups did not like the proposed compromise and engaged in intense lobbying efforts against it. The labor unions strongly objected to limiting public financing to catastrophic medical needs and mandating an expansion of private insurance. Organizations representing health providers objected to the proposed, new, federal catastrophic program and the compulsory aspects and financial regulations in both the employer and catastrophic plan.

The committee was able to reach tentative agreements on some of the less controversial features of the proposal. On the issue of the financing mechanism, however, it split down the middle, reflecting the polarized position of the interest groups. By a 12 to 12 vote the committee rejected a motion to substitute the voluntary, tax-credit approach advocated by the American Medical Association for the financing arrangements in the compromise proposal. On this vote, the 5 southern Democrats on the committee voted with the 7 Republicans in support of the AMA-backed plan. Later, the financing provisions in the mandated, private-insurance part of the proposal were approved by 12 to 11 on a show-of-hands vote.

On August 21, after an hour of heated debate, Mills interrupted the debate and told the committee, "I have never worked harder to reach a consensus than I have on national health insurance. I introduced the Nixon Administration bill with Mr. Schneebeli and the compromise bill with Senator Kennedy. I think the Members of the Committee will agree we have done everything we can to bring about a consensus. We don't have that consensus, and I will not go to the House floor with a Committee bill approved by a 13 to 12 vote."[30] He ended committee deliberations on NHI.

The most recent attempt in Congress to approve health-insurance legislation was in early 1975. With unemployment at the highest level since the depression of the 1930s, there was a push to enact legislation providing health-insurance protection for jobless workers who lose their employment-connected, private-health insurance when they become employed.[31] Initially, the AFL-CIO, American Hospital Association, American Medical Association, Group Health Association of America, Health Insurance Association of America, and the United Auto Workers united in support of a bill introduced by Senators Kennedy, Williams, Javits, and Schweiker. The bill would have used federal general revenues to continue the premium payments for private health-insurance coverage held by unemployed workers when they were still working. It would have maintained the same coverage an individual had while working, as long as he or she remained eligible for unemployment compensation benefits. According to a *National Journal* report, this unlikely coalition of labor unions, insurance companies, and hospitals united in support of the Kennedy bill because "it offered federal subsidies to health care providers, new business to the insurance companies and a method for unions to protect their unemployed members."[32]

It was a short-lived coalition, however, that divided when the lobbies for the insurance industry shifted their support to an alternative proposal developed by the Health Subcommittee of the House Ways and Means Committee chaired by Representative Dan Rostenkowski of Illinois. The Rostenkowski bill proposed a two-part program: one consisting of temporary measures and the other permanent changes. The temporary provisions would continue the health-insurance benefits an unemployed individual eligible for unemployment insurance had while employed. This would be financed by a temporary tax on group health-insurance premiums paid by insurance companies. The permanent part of the proposal would require employers, within 14 months, to revise their private group health-insurance plans to include coverage for workers who lose their jobs, continuing for as long as they were eligible for unemployment compensation.

This was an ingenious proposal that appeared easy to administer and also responded to the administration's objections to any bill with a significant impact on the federal budget. The permanent part of the proposal, however, mandated an expansion of private health-insurance benefits, which was at least conceptually consistent with the national health-insurance proposals sponsored by insurance companies, hospitals, and other conservative groups, strongly opposed by the labor unions and liberal health organizations. In spite of Rostenkowski's contention that his bill was "an interim solution" that did not "commit us to any particular approach to national health insurance," it was perceived by many participants as a step toward national health insurance in the form of putting in place a piece of the plan supported by the insurance industry and health providers. As a result, it interjected the concerns and polarization of NHI politics. The reasons given by the insurance companies for shifting their support to the Rostenkowski bill revealed the traditional split over government versus private financing of medical care. As Lawrence Cathles, Jr., a senior vice-president of Aetna Life and Casualty, explained:

Personally, I think it [the Rostenkowski bill] is by far the best thing that has come down the pike. . . . The thing I worried about under the Kennedy bill was the use of government financing. . . . It would bring in another sizeable bloc of the population whose health insurance needs are paid for by the government. True, he [Kennedy] uses private insurors to administer the program, but this is not inconsistent with the position he took under the Mills-Kennedy health insurance bill. That is, a plan that places private carriers in the role of fiscal intermediaries, but it is *financed and thus controlled* entirely by the government. But the Rostenkowski approach gets away from all of that.[33] [emphasis added]

Because of their opposition to the expension of private-insurance coverage required under permanent provisions, the labor unions persuaded House Speaker Carl Albert to refer the Rostenkowski bill to the House Interstate and Foreign Commerce Committee, which had jurisdiction over the Kennedy bill in the House. Several weeks later the Rogers Subcommittee reported out a bill that retained the temporary part of the Rostenkowski bill, dropped the permanent provisions entirely, and added Medicaid coverage for jobless workers on unemployment compensation who had no health insurance while working.

At this point, the movement to enact an emergency health-insurance bill for the unemployed quickly dissipated, but not because unemployment was decreasing or because any of the problems at which it was aimed had disappeared. It died, partly because the administration was opposed to any bill and partly because it became entangled in a jurisdictional dispute between two House committees, but primarily because the issue had shifted to the locus of the financial operations under national health insurance, and the major advocates of emergency action split over the ideological and economic concerns that have consistently polarized them.

These and less recent attempts to enact health legislation suggest certain conditions that are necessary for the passage of health-insurance legislation. They were met in 1965 when Medicare and Medicaid were enacted and are summarized by Marmor:

The electoral outcome of 1964 guaranteed the passage of legislation on medical care for the aged. Not one of the obstacles to Medicare was left standing. In the House, the Democrats gained thirty-two new seats, giving them a more than two-to-one ratio for the first time since the heyday of the New Deal. In addition,

President Johnson's dramatic victory over Goldwater could be read as a popular mandate for Medicare. The President had campaigned on the promise of social reforms—most prominently Medicare and federal aid to education—and the public seemed to have rejected decisively Goldwater's alternatives of state, local, and private initiative.

Within the Congress, immediate action was taken to prevent the use of delaying tactics previously employed against both federal aid to education and medical care bills. Liberal Democratic members changed the House rules so as to reduce the power of Republican-Southern Democratic coalitions on committees to delay legislative proposals. The twenty-one-day rule was reinstated, making it possible to dislodge bills from the House Rules Committee after a maximum delay of three weeks.

At the same time changes affecting the Ways and Means Committee were made which reduced the likelihood of further efforts to delay Medicare legislation. The traditional ratio of three members of the majority party to two of the minority party was abandoned for a ratio reflecting the strength of the parties in the House as a whole [to-to-one]. In 1965, that meant the composition of Ways and Means shifted from fifteen Democrats and ten Republicans to seventeen Democrats and eight Republicans, insuring a pro-Medicare majority. A legislative possibility until the election of 1964, the King-Anderson program had become a statutory certainty. The only question remaining was the precise form the health insurance legislation would take.[34]

Because of the polarized nature of the conflict among interest groups and members of Congress, it takes a Democratic majority of about 295 in the House and 65 to 70 in the Senate, and a Democratic president interested in health, to enact government financed health-insurance legislation.

There have been important developments in recent years with implications for both the prospects and substance of future health-insurance legislation. The 1974 elections increased the Democratic membership in the House of Representatives from 248 to 290, and thereby reduced the strength of the "conservative coalition" (Republicans plus conservative southern Democrats) from approximately 260 to 215. Fifty-six of the legislators who had sponsored the AMA's national health-insurance proposal in the previous Congress retired or were defeated in 1974. Many of them were replaced by legislators with closer ties to labor and other liberal health groups and less inclined to embrace the AMA's or other conservative organizations' positions on NHI. As shown in table 7-11, the 94th Congress (particularly the House) is more Democratic than any previous Congress since that of 1964, the Congress that enacted Medicare and Medicaid. The possibility of congressional approval of liberal health legislation should be improved as a result of this increased Democratic majority.

Following the 1974 elections a number of organizational reforms were instituted in the House of Representatives that could affect the prospects of NHI legislation. Junior, liberal Democrats, working through the rejuvenated Democratic caucus, deposed three committee chairmen, shifted the committee assignment authority from the Ways and Means Committee to the Steering Committee of the caucus, required all legislative committees to have a 2-to-1

Table 7-11
Party Composition of the House and Senate: 87th to 94th Congresses

Congress	Election Year	House Dems.	House Reps.	Senate Dems.	Senate Reps.
87th	1960	263	174	64	36
88th	1962	258	176	68	32
89th	1964	295	140	67	33
90th	1966	248	187	64	36
91st	1968	243	192	58	42
92nd	1970	255	180	55	45
93rd	1972	243	192	57	43
94th	1974	290	145	61	39

Source: Congressional Research Service, Library of Congress.

plus 1 Democratic majority, and established procedures aimed at opening committee meetings to the public and ensuring freshmen better subcommittee assignments.

The Ways and Means Committee, which prior to the 94th Congress had complete jurisdiction over Medicare, Medicaid, and national health insurance, was changed almost beyond recognition.[35] The size of the committee was increased from 25 to 37, the Democratic majority was increased from 15–10 to 25–12, and over half (19) of the members were new to the committee (including 4 freshmen). Wilbur Mills, who had been chairman of Ways and Means since 1958, was replaced by Al Ullman (D-Ore.). Mills played a major role in the enactment of Medicare and Medicaid in 1965 and was expected to exercise major influence in the design and enactment of national health-insurance legislation.

Ullman does not dominate the agenda-setting and decision-making activities of Ways and Means as did Mills. Ways and Means is not as influential in the House or as responsive to administration positions and proposals as in the past. These changes are due partly to the differences in personality and style of Ullman and Mills, but they are mainly a result of the influx of new members (unaccustomed and unsocialized to the chairman-dominated, consensus-oriented decision-making style under Mills), the increased Democratic majority on the committee and in the House, and the dispersion of power within Ways and Means among senior Democrats who became chairmen of the newly established subcommittees.

Another important change in the House was the shift in jurisdiction over nonpayroll-financed health programs and legislation from the Ways and Means Committee to the Interstate and Foreign Commerce Committee. By 1975 Ways and Means had formally relinquished control over the Medicaid and Maternal and Child Health programs. The debate over health insurance for the unemployed raised the issue of which committee had jurisdiction over national health insurance, but did not resolve it. National health insurance bills are presently being jointly referred to both committees and the health subcommittees of both are moving ahead on national health insurance. The jurisdictional dispute appears to be providing the major incentive for congressional activity on national health insurance at this time, with both subcommittees eager to demonstrate their jurisdictional claims. If not resolved, however, at some later date it could become a major stumbling block to final House action.

The size of the Democratic majority in Congress and the organizational shifts in the House following the 1974 elections are similar to the changes that preceded, and made possible, the enactment of Medicare and Medicaid in 1965. The possibility of congressional approval of government-financed health insurance legislation should be greatly enhanced as a result of these developments. Because of the ideological and political-economic concerns that divide the key groups, and their traditional links to the two parties, however, it is unlikely that any kind of comprehensive, national health-insurance legislation will become law until both the executive and legislative branches are controlled by the same party. Congress is likely to play a major role in the design of future health legislation, but, because of the intense divisions between the major groups, enactment of national health insurance will probably require strong leadership by the president.[36]

The already substantial involvement of the government in health care has important implications for future health legislation. First, the experience under Medicare and Medicaid has demonstrated that we can shift much of the financing of health care from private to public agencies without substantially changing anything else. The changes in direction, distribution, and organization of health care advocated by some proponents of national health insurance will require more than a shift in the bureaucratic location of the primary financial operations, but this might be a necessary first step.

Second, those involved in the administration of existing public programs will most likely be involved in the development and design of future health-insurance programs. Their judgments concerning administrative structures, possibilities, and problems will be influential within the executive agencies and congressional committees responsible for writing health legislation.

Finally, it is highly unlikely that there will be a decrease in government expenditures or regulatory activity. Health care for the elderly, disabled, and poor will very likely remain publicly financed, and the final type of future health-insurance legislation will probably not affect the amount of regulation as much as where the regulating mechanisms are located and the influence of different interests within them. Some form of NHI legislation seems inevitable, and the central legislative issue appears not to be whether but how the government's already substantial role in regulating the health system and assisting individuals to obtain health care should be modified or expanded. That is, the debate seems to have moved beyond whether we should have national health-insurance legislation to what kind: legislation that increases *direct* government regulation and financing of health care or that increases *indirect* government actions such as increasing federal income tax deductions for medical costs, encouraging or mandating the growth of private health-insurance coverage, and increasing regulation and self-regulation in the health industry.

Conclusion

Most commentators assume that pressures on the federal budget preclude immediate comprehensive federal financing of health insurance envisioned by bills such as that of Kennedy-Corman. For this and other reasons, there has resulted a great political interest in plans with high deductibles and/or compulsory employer initiation of plans that spread the cost of the insurance among several parties.[n] Thus, although policy analysis leads to the conclusion that either a direct-cost controlling plan such as the Kennedy-Corman plan or a carefully conceived market-oriented plan such as that proposed by Feldstein is superior to the alternatives, conventional political analysis suggests that an unsatisfactory "middle-ground" solution is probable. Only in the event of an increase in Democratic strength in the legislature *and* the election of a Democratic candidate zealously committed to a plan of the Kennedy-Corman type would the political prediction fail.

---

[n]Some observers have also considered the possibility of phasing in the benefits of the Kennedy-Corman bill by population groups or scope of benefits over a period of years. Because a mixture of private and public financing arrangements would be maintained, a reduced or staged-in federal program would severely limit the operations and effectiveness of the cost-control mechanisms envisioned in the Kennedy-Corman proposal. In fact, until complete coverage is achieved and the cost mechanisms fully implemented, each step toward a universal and comprehensive program could contribute substantially to inflation in health costs. This direction in national policy had not gained significant political support as of this writing; thus, it is not considered in the text. See the discussion of the Scheuer (Child Health Care) bill by Theodore Marmor and Wilbur Cohen before the Health Subcommittee of the House Committee on Interstate and Foreign Commerce, Washington, D.C., June 16, 1976.

8

The Medical Care System under National Health Insurance: Four Models

Walter McClure

I. Introduction and Overview

The burden of this analysis is that the American medical care system will require significant change under any foreseeable form of national health insurance (NHI). Indeed, the medical care system is so central to every issue now pressuring government to intervene in health care that significant change appears unavoidable even in the absence of NHI. With several options available and with such serious consequences for consumers, providers and especially payers of care riding on the decision, the issue of change in the medical care system has received surprisingly little attention in the public debate on NHI. Yet so tightly are the delivery and the financing of medical care interwoven that the fate of NHI and the medical care system are inextricably tied; decisions on either will determine the shape and success of both. Therefore, in asking what kind of NHI we want, Americans might best begin asking what kind of future medical care system we want. They are the same question.

The kind of medical care system we get will result from a complex interplay of both technical and political dynamics. This analysis will examine both to indicate why change seems inevitable, what choices we have and, more speculatively, where our present course may lead.

The issue of medical care system change can be put in the form of a dilemma. On the one hand our society has shifted substantially in the last decade to the idea that health care is a right. We increasingly believe that medical care use should be determined not by income and personal circumstance but by some standard of medical need, and that no one should be bankrupted by ruinous medical expense. We have already made—perhaps without wholly realizing all that was involved—significant, irreversible commitments to this idea through Medicare and Medicaid, and of course we are now contemplating national health insurance.

Reprinted from *Journal of Health Politics, Policy and Law,* 1 (1): 22-68. Copyright 1976 by the Department of Health Administration, Duke University.

This analysis is part of the work carried out by InterStudy under a Health Services Research Center grant from the National Center for Health Services Research. Department of Health, Education and Welfare (Grant No. HS 00471-06). . . . . I would like to thank Gary Appel, Alain Enthoven, William Hsaio, Ted Marmor, Carl Stevens and Bruce Vladeck for their very helpful comments on this paper. They are exonerated from all conclusions and errors of commission and omission herein, which are solely mine.

On the other hand, and here is the dilemma, we already know how to practice a style of medicine in the United States which, if we were to extend it equally to all, would be far more expensive than this nation would or should pay, and far more expensive than the meager improvement to the nation's health would justify. Moreover, the ability of inventive American science and technology to elaborate this style and make it more costly is almost endless. It appears that this costly elaboration is already occurring under Medicare, Medicaid and comprehensive private insurance, to such an extent that government has felt compelled to intervene more and more strongly in the medical care system.

It is our central contention, first, that this cost escalation is unlikely to abate. It is deeply rooted in the structure and incentives of the present medical care system and its financing, and on its own the system has no adequate mechanisms to cope with it. Second, while government may waver on its other health care goals—financial protection of patients, more equitable access, improved effectiveness—it can not afford to waver on cost containment. Caught in a troubled economy between a squeeze on public budgets from other pressing priorities, and footing 40 percent of the rapidly rising health care bill (presently in excess of $100 billion), government will do everything and anything it must to control health care costs. It will not succeed without significant change in the medical care system.

The deep-rooted nature of cost escalation and its seriousness in our present system can be illustrated by an argument and an example. The argument is as follows: As a nation we are increasingly shifting health care from a market to a merit good. Our principle mechanisms for doing so—tax breaks for employment health benefits,[1] Medicare, Medicaid—have resulted in the widespread provision of private and subsidized public health insurance. In effect we heavily reduce the effective price to the patient at the time of service, and commit a third party—the insurer or government—to reimburse the provider for the expense of covered services. This lowering of effective price raises demand.[2] With perhaps over half the population presently covered by good comprehensive insurance,[3] it can be argued the nation is in a state of unsatiated demand. This does not mean that insured consumers are knocking down physician doors; it does mean they would accept more elaborate care if providers recommend or provide it to them. With price and demand no longer the arbiter, the cost and quantity of services delivered becomes determined largely by the supply system, the medical care system. But as our later analysis will attempt to demonstrate, the quantity, quality, style, and therefore cost of medical care can be escalated almost indefinitely, and the present medical care system has every incentive—ethical, professional, financial, and legal—to escalate them. Moreover we as patients support them in this.

The following example shows the seriousness of the results. It is estimated by some medical experts that up to 4 million persons are potentially candidates for coronary bypass graft surgery, an expensive new procedure costing from

$7000-$10,000.[4] No controlled clinical trials to test its efficacy have been performed; but for some patients it is thought to prolong life at least somewhat, for many it relieves pain (although less costly medical treatment may be equally effective in some cases) and for others the benefits have yet to be established.[5] The incidence of the procedure is growing rapidly, apparently constrained mainly by the number of surgeons trained in the operation. If insurance makes price no longer an issue, and the patient's physician recommends the procedure, the patient is unlikely to resist. Thus in the near future the nation could spend up to $20 billion, and thereafter incur annual expenditures of from $2-4 billion, on this one procedure alone if all patients had comprehensive coverage. Even under present coverage at least half that sum will be spent.

Now if one had $20 billion dollars to spend on the health and well-being of the American people, would he choose to spend it on a single procedure of unestablished efficacy? Would he choose to spend it on more medical care alone, even on procedures of established efficacy? Many other non-medical interventions—nutrition, environmental clean-up, traffic safety—improve health; it would seem to be a matter of priorities, of weighing the costs and benefits. The point is, that under present third party reimbursement insurance, one has no choice. If the medical care system elects to perform coronary bypass surgery, the third parties are committed to reimbursing however much they do. And this example, while perhaps more dramatic than most, can be endlessly multiplied.[6]

Thus health care is no longer a benign issue. If we simply continue extending third party insurance coverage without attention to the response of the medical care system, we run the risk of our medical care system becoming a kind of vast vacuum cleaner, sucking uncontrollable amounts of GNP and scarce tax dollars—urgently needed for other equally pressing national priorities—and putting them to medical care. This would seem to be the principal danger facing national health insurance. Should NHI force us to overspend for medical care, the health and well-being of the nation may actually be reduced.

Providers of medical care cannot be blamed for this situation. It is society who changed the rules; it is we the people who are establishing health care as a right. Until the last decade or so, we were content with our medical care system and with health care as a market good. Our expectations have changed. But the structure and incentives of the medical care system have not changed, and cannot cope with health care as a merit good. Thus the problem is structural rather than conspiratorial. It is not that providers will try to do us ill; it is that they will try to do us too much good. And when someone else foots the bill, we will all want the very best. The system is therefore doing exactly what society rewards it to do. If we want health care as a right at a price the nation is willing to pay, we shall not only have to change our medical care system and provider attitudes but our attitudes and expectations as patients as well. We shall have to change from a philosophy of "everything for everybody at the lowest sound cost," which we can't afford, to "that which is most effective to all who will benefit within the means society is willing and able to provide."

What options are available to us? Certainly we do not wish to blindly restrain costs in ways that would jeopardize the health of the American people or impair the effectiveness of our medical care system. Rather, the objective is to contain cost in ways which at the same time improve the efficiency of the system—e.g., health produced per dollar expended—so that effectiveness is maintained or increased. Fortunately, this objective appears possible, though difficult. As suggested in Section III below, there is evidence of sufficient slack in the present medical care system that, by encouragement of more efficient organization and styles of practice, it seems quite possible that medical care costs can be significantly controlled without threat to the nation's health. Experience and research suggest three principal devices with at least the potential to reasonably control costs and encourage efficiency. These three devices, alone or in combination, have very different and significant implications for the future of the medical care system. The nation thus has very genuine choices, representing a range of values and methods. The three devices distinguish themselves according to whether cost-control is exercised primarily through consumers, providers or government:

Consumer Cost-Sharing. The consumer is asked to pay a greater share of the price at the time of service (e.g., deductibles, coinsurance and co-payments). This involves the least change in the medical care system, but to achieve adequate financial protection for catastrophic exepnse, some change will be required. However, cost-sharing of the magnitude necessary to work effectively involves taking away existing benefits, which is extremely difficult politically.

Restructuring the Private System. This would be done in such a way that providers would have improved organization and incentives to accomplish national goals; the encouragement of HMOs and other alternative delivery systems is an example. However, it will require considerable private initiative to create sufficient change to influence the entire medical care system behavior. Encouraging the necessary motivation and acceptance will be difficult.

Public Utility Contols. Experience suggests the controls must be extremely powerful to work. We shall argue that such controls are unlikely to work well until the government can fix the budget for regulated services in advance. Regulatory intervention is the simplest device to implement incrementally, but controls of the magnitude necessary to work effectively will also substantially change the medical care system and will be a long, difficult course politically.

These three devices can be combined in a number of ways to form various future models for the medical care system. Models emphasizing the first two devices may be termed "consumer market" oriented, for they seek to restore market discipline presently lacking in the private system while minimizing government intervention. Models emphasizing regulatory controls accept strong, continuing government intervention, and may be termed "public utility" oriented. In the analysis we shall examine two models of each kind which are likely to work (and one of each kind likely to fail). It will be seen that each medical care system model places different constraints on the design of a national health insurance plan, and conversely, the national health insurance plan influences the direction of change in the medical care system.

Thus national health insurance may offer an opportunity; it can provide the levers to move the medical care system where we want it to go. However, there is little public consensus presently where we want the system to go, indeed there is little awareness that significant change will be needed. In a recent television forum on NHI, only Congressman Ullman insistently recognized the point that the delivery system needs change; the other congressional and administration speakers largely ignored it.[7] Given that all the workable choices appear difficult and will deeply affect all of us, surely the issue needs broad, informed, searching public debate. What kind of medical care system do we want that can provide adequate, effective health care to all at a price the nation can afford?

The analysis is laid out as follows: The next section looks at the goals and problems for national health insurance and the medical care system, and the pressure on the federal government to resolve them. Section III analyzes the underlying causes in the medical care system responsible for these problems. Section IV analyzes the general options available to address these underlying causes and the prospects to implement each option. Finally, Section V speculates where our present course may lead.

II. Problems and Goals for National Health Insurance

Most Americans would probably agree on the following four goals for NHI, if not necessarily on the means to get there. Indeed these are the problems and goals of health policy more generally.

Goal 1. Financial Protection of People from Undue Medical Expense

The United States remains one of the few industrialized countries where an individual can be bankrupted by medical expense. Presently approximately 10 percent of U.S. households spend directly (i.e., excluding employer or other contributions) in excess of 15 percent of their income annually for health insurance premiums and out-of-pocket medical bills.[8] Almost 4 percent spend more than 25 percent of income on such expenses. This burden falls most heavily on the sick and poor. The country must make a decision on whether, how and how much this burden should be shared more widely with the well and the well-off.

Goal 2. More Equitable Distribution of Health Care among the Population

Through Medicare and Medicaid the United States has made enormous strides in improving the distribution of health care by income. In 1963 the poorest third of the population received substantially less services than the highest third. By 1969 both groups used on average about the same amount of services.[9] The price paid in medical cost inflation to accomplish this was substantially more than anticipated. Nevertheless, substantial inequities, by income and area, appear disguised in these averages. Relative to health needs, which are higher among low income persons, the lowest income third of the population should probably be using more services than the rest of the population.[10] Further, the great variation in availability of services creates considerable disparities in per capita use both regionally and locally.[11]

Goal 3. Improved Effectiveness of Health Care

Except for certain underserved groups in the population, it is doubtful that at our present service levels more health care will make measurable improvement in national health levels. Western nations vary more than 200 percent in per capita expenditures for health care but by less than 5 percent in most health indices,[12] and health indices do not particularly correlate with expenditures.[13] Genetics, personal lifestyle, nutrition, environment all appear to play a more determinative role in health than does health care. Nevertheless, the rather meager research on actual patient outcomes of health care in practice suggests there is great variability in effectiveness.[14] Within the limits that health care can achieve, improved effectiveness would provide high health value per dollar of health care.

Goal 4. Control of Health Care Costs

From 1965 to 1975 (fiscal year), per capita health care expenditures in the United States rose from $170 to $476, and total health care expenditures rose from 5.9 percent to 8.3 percent of GNP.[15] Health care is perhaps the largest sector of the economy to sustain such high continued cost escalation. This escalation is particularly troublesome because, although the use of services has increased and is more equitably distributed, it is difficult to find more than marginal improvement in health levels. (It should be noted that during the years 1972 to 1974, health care expenditures remained roughly constant at 7.7 percent of GNP. However, it should also be noted that the annual increase in health care expenditures did not slow down so much as the rest of the badly inflating economy caught up. The analysis of this paper suggests there are many pressures at work in the health care sector likely to continue this cost escalation, even as inflation in the rest of the economy slows down.) In addition to the above goals, there are two additional corollary constraints which NHI should observe:

Constraint 1. Minimal or at Least Evolutionary Disruption of Existing Institutions

Congress tends to move in a cautious incremental way, building on previous actions. Not only is there considerable political inertia in attempting to drastically change large systems of people, such as the health care and health insurance systems, there is considerable danger of confusion and ineffectiveness in doing so. There are also often unforeseen side effects. For example, what might happen to the private financial investment structure of the country should the private health insurance industry be substantially altered? (This is not an argument that it should or should not be in time, only that in a sector as large as health care, drastic change should only be made if necessary, and then at a pace that the nation can politically and practically absorb.) Thus it is probably politically and practically unrealistic to expect enactment of an NHI proposal which goes too far too fast, irrespective of its merits.

Constraint 2. Feasibility, Both of the NHI Plan and Its Implementation Strategy

Any NHI plan must be acceptable to the public and workable in practice. Further, there must be a feasible way to implement the plan, a change strategy to get there from here. These are not the same thing. The analysis of this paper suggests that the NHI proposals most likely to meet the above goals, could they be implemented, are the most difficult to implement. Conversely, the plans most easily implemented are the least likely to fulfill the goals.

To achieve the above goals, an NHI plan will have to specify five issues or "variables:"

Eligibility. Who will be covered? Will eligibility be universal or limited to special groups, will coverage be compulsory or voluntary?

Benefits. Will benefits be basic only, catastrophic only, or comprehensive? Will benefits be uniform or vary among those covered?

Financing. How will the cost of the plan be spread over consumers (via premiums and co-payments), dedicated taxes (payroll tax, surtax and general revenue?

Administration. Shall the plan be publicly or privately administered? In particular, will all private insurers participate or only a limited number, or none? Will they act as underwriters, or as intermediaries only?

Medical care system. What kind of medical care system do we want that can provide equitably distributed, effective health care to all within the means society wishes to pay? What kinds of incentives and controls will create such performance?

Now even superficial inspection shows that all the problems and the goals listed above, even how much financial protection we can afford, crucially depend on the behavior of the medical care system "variable." In the next section we will show just how interrelated and deep-rooted this dependence is. Thus the medical care system is a central issue in the whole NHI question, and indeed of health policy generally.

More particularly, all these goals—and all our other social priorities: welfare, criminal justice, housing, jobs, etc.—depend on having dollars available. Thus the central goal that enables all the rest is cost containment. Yet medical care is the third largest (after debt and Social Security) and fastest growing uncontrollable cost item in the federal budget. This has become particularly critical lately. Before 1972 federal revenues regularly rose faster than committed program expenses because of the natural increase in personal and business incomes. New programs could be financed out of this natural increase in revenue. Since 1972 this situation has begun to reverse, so that commitments are rising faster than revenue[16] (inflation has provided a partial and unwelcome respite). The government has had to raise taxes just to honor present commitments, and cut back programs. Social programs and defense have been the chief casualties. Thus the achievement of a successful NHI program, which does not devour scarce dollars needed for other equally important national priorities, depends upon the achievement of a medical care system with reasonably controllable costs.

To make things more difficult, all the "variables" above are highly interrelated. The Congress cannot answer them independently one-by-one without getting highly contradictory, conflicting policy. If the desired medical care system of the future is specified, the remaining variables are to a large degree determined or at least constrained. Conversely, if the other variables—eligibility, benefits, financing and administration—are specified, they will largely determine, intentionally or unintentionally, the future medical care system. Thus the nation has an extremely complex decision-making process to go through. If it chooses the other "variables" unmindful of the medical care system, it may wind up with a system that won't hold costs. And it may find it difficult and expensive to undo and redo these unmindful decisions.

It is particularly disturbing, then, that the medical care system has received so little attention in the current debate on NHI. Few of the major NHI proposals seriously address the problem of a coherent medical care system strategy, and make token recognition of cost control with piecemeal measures for which there is little evidence of effectiveness, either in this or other countries.[17] In the absence of debate, the public appears to be under the illusion that through NHI they can achieve (1) complete financial protection and (2) controlled costs, and (3) still retain the present system and style of health care while (4) improving access to service into the bargain. This analysis will suggest at best we can achieve any three of these desires but not the fourth: either we shall make substantial change in our health care system, or we shall suffer runaway costs, or we shall considerably lower our sights on the goals specified above. At worst, all of these events may occur.

III. An Analysis of Medical Care System Behavior

This section attempts to show that the major problems outlined in the previous section do not lend themselves to quick band-aid solutions but are deeply rooted in the structure and incentives of the present medical care system and its financing. We shall try to identify the basic structure and incentive elements determining system behavior, so that the policy and political analyst can understand what needs change and anticipate how the system will respond to various corrective strategies under NHI.

Ideally we would prefer a rigorous general theory of medical care system behavior, but such a theory is probably still some years off. However, recent research has uncovered many bits and pieces of the puzzle which, combined with plausible assumptions and arguments, can be woven into an analysis providing at least qualitative understanding of gross system behavior important to policy. With the caveat that conceptual analysis is not a substitute for a quantitative theory, we shall advance such an analysis.

The analysis is developed as follows. We start with a fundamental assumption, that the behavior of organized systems of people is determined by the structure and incentives of the system. We then set forth as further basic assumptions—generalizing from research, observation and experience—what we believe to be the key structural and incentive factors governing the behavior of the medical care system. While we shall attempt to make these generalizations plausible by explanation and example, we shall not primarily defend them directly. Rather we shall treat the assumptions as postulates, to be justified by their ability to rationally explain or predict system behavior confirmed or consistent with research findings. (If we are unable to plausibly deduce important known system behavior, this would indicate either error in the basic assumptions or that additional important structural and incentive factors have been overlooked. On the other hand, if most of the important behavior of the system can be accounted for, we gain confidence that the basic assumptions must be part of any eventual theory of the medical care system.) Once we have reasonably justified the basic assumptions in this manner, we shall use them in later sections to infer medical care system response to various policy proposals and NHI plans. Of course, our deductions will be based on rational argument rather than rigorous derivation, and the farther we stray from confirmed behavior, the more speculative the analysis becomes. Nevertheless this type of structure-incentive analysis is believed a useful tool deserving wider application for the policy analyst working with social systems generally, and may serve as a source of hypotheses for an eventual, more rigorous theory.

A. Basic Assumptions

1. *The medical care system behaves the way it is structured and rewarded to behave. Policy strategies will succeed or fail depending on how they address or alter the basic structure and incentives producing present system behavior.* This assumption is asserted as self-evident. By structure is meant the nature of the individuals and organizational elements in the system and the relationships among them. By incentives is meant all the positive and negative rewards and penalties—personal, social, professional, financial, legal—operating on individuals and organized elements in the system.

2. *The quality, quantity and style*[18] *of medical care are indefinitely expansible. The medical care system can legitimately absorb every dollar society will make available to it.* The nature of a system's product is one of the most important structural elements. In the case of the medical care system, the probabilistic and uncertain nature of both health and medical science implies that medical need is virtually inexhaustible. Providers can always try to provide ever greater safety margins for treatable patients, treat more and more hopeless patients, and screen for less and less probable diagnoses. For example, why perform $50 of laboratory tests to be 95 percent sure of a diagnosis, if $250 of tests will provide 97 percent certainty? Or, if a patient's condition is otherwise hopeless, why not perform an operation with a one in a thousand chance of success? Or, if an annual physical is good, why isn't a semi-annual physical better? Physicians already give themselves and their families 30 percent more care than the national average,[19] and inventive American science and technology can endlessly elaborate the possibilities. While the medical care system is too large and complex to respond instantaneously, eventually the final check on what gets done is the dollars available.

Elaborate medical care is not necessarily bad nor unnecessary (and consequently will not be curtailed by controls aimed at bad or unnecessary care), but it does rapidly run up against the law of diminishing marginal returns. The first few dollars invested in medical care—for immunizations, setting broken bones, etc.—are very effective in improving health. But it becomes increasingly more difficult and expensive to make similar health gains as we spend more.

Beyond a certain point all the additional tests provide little extra safety margins, the heroic measures only prolong the coma and postpone the inevitable, and medical care even begins to produce complications from its own complex interventions.[20]

3. *The incentives on providers in the present medical care system are powerfully skewed toward specialized, technological, high cost care.* The following examples illustrate some of these incentives. Peer reputation is a powerful motivator in most professions, and the physician gains far greater peer (and public) prestige practicing highly-specialized, technological care than practicing general primary medicine.[21] Financially, specialty work returns significantly greater income per hour than primary care,[22] and fee-for-service rewards the provision of more services and more expensive services.[23] Educationally, the physician is trained in medical centers engaging in highly specialized secondary and tertiary care, presenting role models he will be professionally socialized and rewarded to follow. Ethically the provider is bound to do all he can for each patient he accepts. Legally, physicians feel that malpractice doctrine seems to assert that, in event of an untoward result, the physician had better be able to demonstrate he performed all standard (whatever the court defines this to be) procedures even if he believes them excessive and unwarranted. Thus, unless altered or checked by limited financing, these incentives should lead physicians toward elaborate, specialized, high style practice which helps the few at great great expense rather than lower cost, lower style medicine which helps the many.

4. *The widespread extent of private and public third-party reimbursement health insurance, well over half of which appears quite comprehensive, provides almost open-ended financing to the medical care system.* The patient (first party) and provider (second party) control the cost and use of services, but the bill is paid by a third party—the insurer—who is committed to reimburse whatever covered services are done. The consumer, once his premium has been paid (and to the extent that he does not have to pay additional co-payments at the time of the service), has every incentive to receive benefits that may help him, the provider has every incentive to render them. The insurer, public or private, risks the wrath of both the consumer and providers if he interferes. To control expenditures under third-party reimbursement health insurance, the insurer would have to intervene in virtually every individual medical transaction to judge its costs and appropriateness, a questionable role for a financial agent and a task which not even public insurers have succeeded at. (Thus Canada with universal public health insurance of the third-party reimbursement type has cost escalation comparable to the United States with its mixed public-private insurance system,[24] even though Canada has tried virtually every control proposed for the United States.) With an estimated 80-90 percent of Americans having at least some public or private health insurance, and well over half rather comprehensively covered,[25] the medical care system has almost a blank check for its activities.

5. *The medical care system is fragmented into many small, independent units of production—predominantly solo physicians—inhibiting economies of scale and continuity, and creating strong externalities among the units.* By externalities is meant that costs and savings are not borne by the provider who creates them. For example, because physicians and hospitals are independent, the physician does not bear the cost of the hospital or its specialized facilities when he places a patient there. For example, the good family practitioner who detects and treats an illness early receives payment only for a few office calls; he receives none of the hundreds of dollars saved from the operation he may have prevented thereby. (These externalities tend to be reinforced by the consumer, who is far more motivated to seek care for late stage illness than for early stage, asymptomatic conditions.) Thus the present fragmented system, itself a product of historical structure and incentive forces, now acts to produce both structural inhibition and an absence of financial incentives to use the mix of health resources efficiently

6. *The consumer is a poor judge of either the effectiveness or efficiency of his medical care nor is he able to get much information about them, giving the provider considerable latitude over the type and quantity of services demanded.* The consumer seeks health. He receives health services, about which he knows little and, under present professional controls, can obtain little objective information on cost or quality.[26] His information costs are therefore high and increase with the complexity of the episode, complicated by the presence of illness itself. He can of course judge expense (and may often, incorrectly, equate it with quality, and has several means to regulate his demand if he feels the benefit of health care unlikely to justify the expense: by not presenting himself for treatment, by non-compliance, by pressuring the provider for alternative cheaper treatment, or by seeking second opinions and alternative providers. The latter means are partially biased by professional control (as well as present malpractice doctrine) over standards of practice: for example, it is hard to imagine an American obstetrician recommending home delivery by a midwife, though the Dutch experience suggests that, properly organized, this can be quite as safe and much less expensive for uncomplicated deliveries as our specialized hospital delivery.[27] Were quality assured by other means and if objective information were available, price pressure could make consumers a more effective force for efficiency, but with the artificially low prices created by insurance, consumer choice is a poor force for either effectiveness or efficiency.

7. *The medical care system has no ongoing mechanism to systematically monitor patient outcomes, nor is any provider accountable for the patient's health beyond the services that provider rendered.* The medical care system has little knowledge of nor accountability for its final product: health. For example, if a health survey found an excessive amount of uncontrolled high blood pressure in a community, what could it do with such information; no provider can be held accountable either for the problem or its correction. Each provider can choose the type of service he shall render, and is not responsible for other health

problems in the population no matter how pressing. Moreover, once the provider has completed an episode of services, he tends to lose track of the patient. There is neither mechanism nor incentive to determine that the patient received all additional services of other providers to assure that his health was optimized. When a system is without feedback or accountability for goals, that system will tend to confuse means with ends. If the medical care system does not measure its productivity in terms of health, it will measure productivity in terms of services and dollars, even though these correlate only weakly with health.[28] Thus the system will tend to maximize on services rather than on health.

B. Inferences Concerning Medical Care System Behavior

We shall now attempt to justify the above structure and incentive assumptions by showing they provide a rational explanation of gross medical care system behavior and in particular the problems outlined in Section II. We shall draw inferences on system behavior from the assumptions and document that the inference is confirmed or consistent with research findings.

1. The medical care system will likely be subject to strong provider induced demand-pull cost escalation. Because of the reduced out-of-pocket price, the heavily insured consumer will accept a more expensive level of care (assumption 4), which allows providers to follow their powerful incentives (assumption 3) to practice more elaborate styles of care (assumption 2). It is important to note that expenditures should escalate not because the cost of inputs pushes them up (cost-push), but because insurance permits providers to increase prices and services and put the dollars into more costly inputs (demand-pull). As noted in the overview, we emphasize that in medical care this "demand"-pull is not simple consumer demand (there are no patient queues to speak of), but includes substantial provider induced demand made possible by insurance; the consumer himself does not demand high style medical care, but if insurance removes the restraining effect of price, the consumer will largely accept what his provider recommends. As we have shown, providers have powerful incentives to recommend high style. Expanded coverage under NHI would likely aggravate such cost escalation pressures.

Research Findings. Cost escalation has already been documented in Section II.4. Recent economic research suggests this cost escalation is consistent with predominant demand-pull.[29] Thus a kind of Parkinson's Law of medical care obtains; standards of practice eventually rise to absorb the dollars available.

2. The medical care system will likely be characterized by over-elaborate inefficient, cost-ineffective styles of practice. Such "high style" is not necessarily ineffective; it is simply more expensive and wasteful than more efficient, "lower style" practice patterns that are equally effective in producing health. In other words we expect the system not only to be using increasingly more dollars, but to be using them inefficiently. This inference follows from the absence of incentives for efficiency and the strong incentives for inefficiency (assumptions 3, 4, 5, 6, 7). Expanded coverage under NHI could thus aggravate inefficiency. *Research Findings.* Upon this vital inference rests the case that this nation can contain medical costs without threat to the health of its people. Three types of evidence strongly confirm this inference. First, utilization studies among comparable populations with comparable health indices show utilization of common services, such as hospital days and common surgery, varies by as much as two-fold, indicating the prevalence of inefficient high style practice patterns. Second, controlled clinical trials and outcomes studies suggest that much medical care has little effect, and that lower style clinical methods are often as effective as higher style methods. Third, efficiency studies show that, even beyond inefficiently high utilization, medical resources are used inefficiently.

The most rigorous utilization studies of matched populations compare HMOs (which eliminate externalities and have strong incentives for efficiency, see Section IV, Model 4 below) with traditional fee-for-service providers. Even after adjusting for age, sex and other factors, HMOs use 30–50 percent less hospital days, fewer physicians and 10–30 percent less total cost, per capita.[30] The few comparative studies of patient end-results in matched populations indicate both styles more or less equally effective.[31] Less controlled studies within the traditional system itself show extreme variations in utilization rates by area and region. Lewis[32] found common surgical procedure rates per person varied two-fold across Kansas counties. Similarly, Wennberg et al.[33] found great variations in hospitalization per person across Vermont counties. The national health survey[34] found great variations in hospital use per person among regions of the United States, even for the same procedures; for example, length of stay for uncomplicated delivery was five days in the East, but only three days in the West. These variations appear far too great to be attributed to population differences,[35] and are more likely accounted for by styles and patterns of practice. This is further supported by evidence from controlled, clinical trials and outcomes studies.[36] The evidence suggests not only the common use of procedures of unproven efficacy, but also the tendency of the medical care system to move toward high style procedures, even before their efficacy is fully established, when equally effective but less costly lower style procedures are available. Finally, efficiency studies confirm excessive inefficient use of expensive resources. For example, hospitals operate at inefficient levels of occupancy,[37] suggesting a major surplus of beds and service facilities. In other words, the system not only has inefficiently high utilization, this utilization itself is produced inefficiently. Further studies demonstrating both inefficient styles and inefficient production of services within the traditional system come from pre-admission testing,[38] pre-admission screening,[39] pre-surgical referral,[40] substitution of out-patient for inpatient care,[41] in-hospital review,[42] and others.[43]

This ample evidence of widespread inefficiency confirms our contention that, if we can successfully reduce inefficiency, we can contain medical costs without harm to people's health or the effectiveness of the medical care system. But we shall not accomplish improved efficiency until we alter the structure and incentives in the present medical care system and its financing (listing in Section A above) which have produced and now maintain existing inefficient styles of both medical practice and operation. Such change will be no simple task.

3. The type and use of service in local populations will likely depend much more upon the organization of the medical care system serving that population than upon the characteristics of the population served. From the great latitude in style of medical practice (assumption 2), it can be inferred that in any area with adequate income and insurance levels (assumption 4), providers can make an adequate income providing elaborate care to the few or basic care to the many (assumption 2); providers thus have considerable latitude to choose the type and quantity of service they will provide. Expanded coverage under NHI could give the medical care system even greater latitude over utilization of services.

Research Findings. Evidence supporting this inference comes from the failure of theories of consumer demand to account for much of the variation in utilization,[44] from the large differences in service and resource use among comparable populations cited in point 2 above, particularly between those served respectively by fee-for-service and prepaid group practice and from studies demonstrating supply appears to at least in part generate its own demand.[45]

4. Physicians will tend to increasingly specialize in inefficiently excessive numbers. This inference follows from the powerful incentives to specialize (assumption 3), coupled with the observation that physicians can always find things to do for patients (assumption 2) which patients will accept in the absence of any economic check (assumptions 4 and 6). Expanded coverage under NHI could thus aggravate over-specialization.

Research Findings. The relative increase in specialists and decrease in primary care physicians both in practice and in training is well documented.[46] Evidence that the physician distribution is inefficiently over-specialized comes from comparison with the physician distribution in HMOs,[47] which have strong incentives for efficiency; HMOs produce apparently comparable health results with relatively fewer specialists and relatively more primary physicians than the U.S. average. This result also supports the previous inference, since more specialists will result in proportionately more specialty care.

5. Physicians will tend to be maldistributed by area, with specialists concentrated in professionally attractive areas. Only general and family practitioners are likely to be geographically distributed more evenly. If insurance and income levels are adequate, specialists can concentrate in professionally attractive areas by using their latitude to provide more elaborate services to fewer people.

(Indeed the desire to locate in a professionally attractive but physician-rich area adds one more incentive for physicians to specialize.) There is sufficient flexibility and expansibility in the medical ecology (assumption 2) and enough financing available (assumption 4) that specialists can pretty much avoid competing with each other, even in areas of high specialist concentration, and still maintain incomes. Only general and family practitioners, whose services are not usually covered by insurance, will be under much market pressure to distribute more evenly.[48] Expanded coverage under NHI could thus aggravate geographic maldistribution.

Research Findings. The geographic distribution of physicians is known to be uneven[49] with general practitioners showing a moderately even distribution[50] and specialists concentrated in certain metropolitan areas. There is also some evidence consistent with the above argument that in physician-rich areas on average each physician renders less but more expensive service, and each person receives in total more services, than in physician-scarce areas.[51]

6. Catastrophic care episodes requiring large expenditures should be escalating in cost much more rapidly than all care, and consume an increasing percentage of the health care dollar. This follows from all the incentives for physicians to engage in ever more specialized technological care, coupled with the fact that more and more people are becoming covered by more comprehensive insurance. We can expect this to create a market for medical technology which American science and industry will attempt to fill. Expanded coverage under NHI could thus aggravate catastrophic care escalation.

Research Findings. The best evidence available suggests that in 1970 the top 1 percent of the population with the most expensive episodes consumed roughly 25 percent of all health care dollars, and the expenses of this top 1 percent were escalating 13–18 percent annually compared with about 10 percent for all care.[52] It seems doubtful that this rise can be attributed to increased catastrophic illness; the above explanation seems more likely. Much more research on the incidence, cost and outcomes of catastrophic illness is vitally needed.

The examples above provide some confidence that the basic structure and incentive assumptions in Section A above can plausibly explain gross system performance and are likely to be an important part of any eventual theory of medical care system behavior. These assumptions shall now be applied more speculatively to conditions which may obtain under NHI proposals.

IV. Strategies and Prospects for the Medical Care System Under NHI

In this section we shall ask three questions: What NHI strategies might successfully achieve health care goals, especially cost containment? What is the likely impact of each strategy on the future medical care system? What are the prospects for implementing each strategy?

While an NHI strategy should be capable of achieving each of the major health care goals (Section II), the discussion shall focus on the cost containment issue for three reasons. First, cost containment is central; without it the dollars for the remaining goals will not be there. Second, because of the intimate relation between the medical care system and its financing, cost containment will have the greatest impact on the system. Third, a strategy which does not sufficiently contain costs will be unstable; the nation will keep shifting strategies until cost escalation is held to a tolerable level. Though important in their own right, the other goals—financial protection, equity and effectiveness—would take the discussion too far beyond the scope of this paper, and will be considered only as they limit possible cost containment methods or additionally impact the medical care system.

A. Methods for Cost Containment

The key to medical care system performance apparently lies in its structure and incentives. To determine successful methods for cost containment, we must therefore look at the structure and incentive factors of Section III. A creating cost escalation and inquire what needs to be changed. Two factors appear crucial: first, third party reimbursement health insurance, which creates artificially low prices for the consumer, gives an open-ended commitment to the provider, and allows the third party little control; and second, the powerful cost-raising incentives intrinsic in the present medical care system. To contain costs then, we shall either have to shift much of the payment control function from the poorly positioned third party to other parties better able to control the price and quantity of service, or alter the misdirected incentives in the present medical care system either through internal reforms or external controls, or do both.

If the incentives in the medical care system are not altered, the controls on price and quantity—and the incentives on the controllers to effectively exercise these controls—will have to be correspondingly more powerful.

There are three parties with the potential to control the price and quantity of services: the consumer, the provider, and the government. The major methods for cost containment divide naturally according to which of these three parties assumes control of medical expenses. Strategies for the medical care system (and NHI) will generally combine consistent combinations of all three methods, but may be classified according to which methods are emphasized. The methods may be described as follows:

Consumer Cost-Sharing. This method shifts the risk and control of medical expense more to the consumer, who can presumably best judge the utility of medical care to himself compared to other things he might purchase. The method is based on altering insurance benefits. If insurance removes the direct cost of care from the consumer, he will have every incentive to use all the care offered him. The consumer can presumably be induced to use care more prudently if he is made to share directly some portion of the cost. (He would still be financially protected if his share could not exceed some maximum limit.) Cost-sharing approaches include making the deductible very large ("catastrophic" insurance), or having stiff coinsurance (say 25 percent). Also the consumer could share in the premium. Note that to work effectively, cost-sharing must be simple and uniform. Otherwise the consumer will not know in advance what his cost-share will be when he purchases services. It is doubtful that any consumer knows his cost-share under the present plethora of varying deductibles, coinsurance rates, inside limits, maximum limits and exclusions.

Provider Incentives Approach. This method shifts the risk and control of medical expense more to the providers, who can presumably best decide the necessity and most efficient use of care. It is based on preserving but restructuring the private medical care system to alter the present cost-raising incentives. The best articulated examples of this approach are the so-called HMOs, embracing a wide variety of prepaid comprehensive care organizations competing with traditional providers. Other alternative delivery systems with prepaid comprehensive care arrangements also seem possible but are unproven. Consumers enroll in the organization of their choice and pay a fixed monthly amount for all their care. The amount is set by the HMO in competition with other plans. The combination of comprehensive prepayment directly to providers and competition for consumers reduces incentives for high style and eliminates externalities. Thus these providers must attract and care for their enrollees within a fixed total budget determined by the market, which presumably places upon them a powerful incentive to provide economical, effective care. Even greater savings are presumably possible if HMOs and other alternative systems become prevalent enough to put market pressure on fee-for-service providers. Note that for this approach to work effectively, consumers must bear directly some portion of the premium or be allowed to receive additional benefits out of savings. Otherwise there is no incentive to keep premiums down or choose efficient systems. Other incentive arrangements short of HMOs (such as prospective reimbursement) though still unproven, also seem possible, but appear to require greater public intervention and thus verge more toward the public utility approach below.

Public Utility Approach. This method shifts the control of medical expense more to the government, which presumably has the requisite power and expertise unavailable to consumers and third parties to control costs and improve efficiency.

It is assumed that the government can eventually exercise regulatory controls over the inputs, the process and the outcomes of care in any combination and degree necessary until cost escalation is reduced to a tolerable level. Note that for this approach to work effectively, government control must extend universally over all medical care, not just public programs such as Medicare and Medicaid. Otherwise providers will use their latitude to concentrate on more elaborate care for the middle class, and the controls will simply squeeze the poor and the old or shift their costs to private patients.

In the remainder of this section we shall examine six models of NHI which combine these cost control methods in different ways. We may classify these models into two kinds: those which emphasize the first two methods shall be termed "consumer market" oriented, for they emphasize a private approach to medical care delivery and minimize government intervention. Those which emphasize government regulation shall be termed "public utility" oriented. By examining the incentives on the various parties expected to exercise control, we may analyze how well the models are likely to contain costs.

B. Two Models Likely to Fail

This section analyzes two models, one consumer market oriented and one public utility oriented, which are unlikely to work well.

Model 1. The Present Medical Care System with Universal Third-Party Financing.
This model would leave the present medical care system unchanged, and simply extend present third-party reimbursement insurance to all.

Prospects for Cost Containment. The analysis of Section III suggests this model would simply aggravate every existing problem in the medical care system, particularly cost escalation. Comprehensive, universal third-party insurance wipes out the last vestige of any market discipline in the present system.

Prospects for Implementation. Because the model leaves existing institutions alone, it can be expected to gain much support. However, the model is unstable; it can't last. Runaway costs will force intervention, probably in the form of ever increasing government regulation since the government will be subsidizing much of the bill. This appears to be the lesson of Medicare and Medicaid, which essentially used this model for the poor and the old: if public financing of medical care is expanded without altering the structure and incentives of the delivery system, runaway cost will drag the government ever more deeply into regulation of the delivery system.[53] Nevertheless, since is doubtful that the present strong government entry into health care regulation would have occurred without cost escalation in Medicare and Medicaid, this model may represent one way, albeit a very expensive one, to creat sufficient pressure to make the remaining models more palatable.

Model 2. Public Utility Process Controls with Universal Third-Party Financing. Public utility cost controls in medical care may be divided into two kinds: process controls which try to directly limit the price and quantity of services (such as utilization review, the process medical audit, fee controls, etc.), and input controls which try to limit the manpower, facilities, and total dollars available to provide medical care. This model would extend third party coverage, either private or public, to all and rely on public utility process controls to contain costs.

Prospects for Cost Containment. Our previous analysis (Section III) as well as experience suggest that public utility process controls are unlikely to work well. The great latitude in medical need, the ill-defined nature of health services, and the sheer volume of services rendered suggest the magnitude of the difficulties. Price controls alone will not work, because providers can always increase the quantity and the mix of services (toward higher style), or even redefine the content of services. But to judge the necessity and appropriateness of each service rendered requires not only huge administrative review apparatus (expensive in itself) but strong provider input. And providers have little incentive to make such review work, and great incentive not to make it work.[54] Indeed, process provider review of procedures is as likely to raise costs as lower them[55] since providers will likely equate high style with quality.[56] How will the bureaucracy counter such judgments? Under the best of circumstances public utility regulation is vulnerable to capture by the regulated;[57] to attempt regulation in an area so fraught with medical judgment and ambiguity is to virtually invite it.

Evidence to support the above argument is ambiguous but not inconsistent. Review of such research as exists provides little evidence that process controls make any difference, and some evidence that such effect as they do have may wear off rather quickly.[58] Under Phase II and III of the recent price controls, the experience was that annual service price increases declined from 8 percent to 4 percent,[59] whereas the annual increase in total expenditures only declined from 12 percent to 10 percent[60] (presumably because the quantity and style of services remained uncontrolled). Some of this decline was in evidence before the controls began, perhaps from the recession, so how much can be attributed to the controls is not known. Thus, for a creditable but considerable administrative effort, our most ambitious attempt at price controls, so far, made at most some decrease in the magnitude of the annual cost increase, and whether this could be sustained is problematic.

Prospects for Implementation. The experience of Medicare and Medicaid suggests process controls are among the easier types of public utility regulation to enact. But like the previous model, this model seems unstable. When this model fails to contain costs, government will try successively stronger process controls and eventually move toward strong input controls. (It is already attempting weak input controls on facilities via Certificate of Need laws.) The danger of this incremental approach to strong public utility controls is that it is not only expensive (e.g., we endure cost escalation until this model is supplanted), it may stifle the medical care system with a massive fragmented, bureaucratic, expensive, indifferently effective regulatory apparatus which is unlikely to go away when more effective regulation is found. There is little history of deregulation in this country.

C. Four Models That Might Work

This section analyzes four models—two market oriented and two public utility oriented—that might achieve the NHI goals of Section II. The four models chosen were selected because each emphasizes primarily one of the cost control methods in Section IV. A above. We may thereby gain some insight into further models combining all three methods by extrapolating the analyses for these four.

Model 3. Major Risk-Insurance. This model, articulated by Pauly and by Feldstein,[61] carries consumer cost-sharing to a fine art. The intent is to significantly reduce third-party financing by placing the consumer at substantial risk for the great majority of his care while still absolutely protecting him from bills large relative to his ability to pay. This is accomplished by totally insuring the consumer for all annual medical expenses, the threshold of complete coverage can be raised to say 20 percent or 15 percent. Below this threshold, he must pay all medical expenses out-of-pocket. Alternatively, to give the consumer a cost-share in even larger expenses, the threshold of complete coverage can be raised to say 20 percent of income and a coinsurance rate of 50 percent or 75 percent can be placed on expenses below the threshold, so that again the consumer is never at risk for more than 10 percent or 15 percent of income. Recognizing that for low income persons, even 10 percent of income is onerous, the co-insurance rate and threshold could be proportionately reduced (income related) on a sliding scale according to income in any way deemed equitable.

Prospects for Cost Containment. Evidence tends to support that heavy cost-sharing can effectively control costs. The more carefully price elasticity of medical care is measured, the more elastic it appears to be.[62] (The argument that the physician, not the patient, controls demand appears to be strictly true only in conditions of unsatiated demand created by third-party financing.) Certainly the huge increase in use of services by the poor and old under Medicare and Medicaid show that price has a substantial impact on demand. Thus in principle the degree of cost-sharing can be increased sufficiently to control costs to whatever degree society desires.

A greater concern is that MRI will contain costs at the expense of health, especially of the poor. A thorough discussion of this point is beyond the scope of this paper, but briefly, it seems unlikely that MRI will threaten either health or equity. In principle at least, MRI can be income-related to any degree society desires, eliminating bias against the poor (although too many income-related variations raise questions of administrative feasibility). And if an adequate level of medical care is thereby placed within the ability to pay of every person, there is no reason to think that health should be greatly endangered at our present levels of health care use.[63] If beyond this basic standard, consumers elect to put their money to other things, rather than health care which medical experts deem important, it must be remembered that consumer decisions disturb experts in all fields. It is a question of values; individual choice vs. social concern. If after placing adequate medical care within individuals' ability to pay, society wishes to assure equity beyond what individuals would choose on their own, then the price of equity will be greater intervention in the medical care system.

Prospects for the Medical Care System. MRI affords very complete financial protection to individuals. It also appears able to contain cost, but only below its threshold. This is an extremely important limitation which MRI shares with any cost-sharing approach. If there is to be financial protection, then at some point cost-sharing must be reduced to where it becomes ineffectual. At this point other cost control methods must be used. In the absence of controls yet to be specified, MRI is likely to distort the amount of resources going to secondary and tertiary care routinely rendered above the threshold, precisely the area most vulnerable to cost escalation (see III.B.6).

The problem is significant, and characteristic of any insurance plan covering catastrophic illness. By Feldstein's own estimate, medical care above the MRI threshold presently accounts for more than 30 percent of the health care dollar. But MRI, by offering complete catastrophic coverage, will greatly increase (consumer and provider-induced) demand for catastrophic care, which is only poorly covered now,[64] (and may freeze externalities for such care into the system) and create an excessive market for high cost/low benefit technology that American science and industry will rush to fill. Unless controlled, cost escalation of catastrophic care may significantly offset savings in basic care and continue the present maldistribution by specialty and geographic area (see III.B.5).

This objection is hardly fatal to MRI, and can be resolved by applying other cost control methods, most likely public utility allocation controls (see Models 3 and 4 below), to catastrophic care. The problems in doing this have been touched on elsewhere.[65] However, all these solutions involve important intervention in the medical care system, although rather less than in the models below simply because intervention is restricted to the catastrophic care area. In fact, the infrequent number of episodes which reach catastrophic magnitude may make effective control in this area more feasible than models attempting across the board controls.

Prospects for Implementation. MRI could be administered either publicly or by private insurers. However, in order for the cost containment rationale of MRI to work effectively, MRI must (1) be fairly universal and (2) not be supplemented by basic benefits below the threshold. If some people have comprehensive benefits and some have MRI, it is likely that accepted standards and style of medical practice will be determined under comprehensive coverage (see III.B.3), and MRI will be accused of forcing people to accept second class care. If MRI is supplemented by basic coverage, then the total spectrum of care is covered, and the cost containment rationale of MRI falls apart.

There thus arises considerable political difficulty in implementing MRI. Feldstein[66] believes that MRI would drive out comprehensive health insurance in a competitive situation because it offers complete financial protection at one third the cost of comprehensive insurance. If so, the government need only offer a federal MRI policy (or alternatively mandate that private insurers offer an MRI policy as a dual choice to conventional health insurance), and the market would solve the implementation problem. Such an implementation strategy would be a political godsend, for it requires almost no direct intervention in existing medical and insurance arrangements. Unfortunately there is little evidence that it would work. The evidence from Medicare and group insurance is that individuals will purchase supplementary insurance against deductibles and co-insurance even for very comprehensive policies;[67] and it is unlikely that labor, which bargains for much of the group health insurance market, will consent to give up basic benefits already won. In at least one instance, MRI in a dual choice situation with conventional benefits was almost totally rejected by a university faculty.[68] Further resistance may come from the insurance industry, whose revenues would be drastically reduced under MRI.

Thus the only recourse to implement MRI would appear to be requiring by legislation that no other kind of health insurance could be sold. This seems politically impossible at this time. It would require taking away the great bulk of existing benefits, and there is no example of a country which has been able to successfully remove even modest benefits more than temporarily.[69] Imagine the politician or labor leader who must report to his constituency that he has just given up all their basic health benefits!

In sum, MRI supplemented by catastrophic care controls appears to be a very promising option which creates the least interference in the medical care system, but there is no simple way to get from here to there. A great deal of public information, debate and understanding would be necessary to make this option palatable.

Model 4. Alternative Delivery Systems Competing under Universal Coverage. This model was first articulated by Ellwood et al.[70] as a general strategy for restructuring the private medical care system to contain cost and improve equity and effectiveness. Its application under various national health insurance plans has been discussed by McClure[71] (although national health insurance is not a prerequisite to implementing the strategy). This approach stresses the provider incentives cost containment method above, with the idea that if the structure and incentives of the private medical care system can be properly set, the system will work out the myriad details to achieve public goals on its own without the necessity of detailed government involvement. The model would stimulate a variety of directly prepaid comprehensive medical care organizations with improved structure and incentives, competing with each other and traditional providers. Under universal coverage, people are entitled to federally specified health care benefits and receive an income-related subsidy or voucher to purchase them. The voucher may be applied to any of several qualified plans—whether one of the new alternative systems or a conventional third party insurance plan (public or private) using traditional providers—which compete on price and extra benefits. The consumer pays the difference between the value of his voucher and the price of the plan he chooses, so that consumers and plans face market discipline.

Prospects for Cost Containment. Both analysis and research evidence suggest this model might contain costs and encourage efficiency if it can be implemented. In the new alternative systems consumer choice, direct prepayment to providers, and the elimination of externalities provide new incentives for efficient, effective care. Prepayment direct to the provider organization rather than a third party compels the provider to work from a fixed budget so that he must be cost conscious. Because it is comprehensive, the provider organization can capture the savings from reduced use of hospital and specialty care and apply them to primary care. And because the consumer has a choice, the provider organization must continually strive to satisfy him, nor can it arbitrarily raise its price (capitation). Consumer choice itself is strengthened because the consumer does not make decisions on individual services but rather on an entire comprehensive care organization, which is large enough that he can get information from several of his neighbors. (More objective information along the lines of "Truth in Health Care Coverage" could also be made available.) And he makes his decisions in advance, uncomplicated by the presence of illness. The broadening of consumer choice to include new alternative systems further implies that traditional providers will now also have to offer more economical care in order to compete for consumers.

Evidence tending to confirm the above arguments is of three kinds. First, existing mature HMOs show savings averaging 10–30 percent over traditional providers while achieving equally effective results.[72] Second, while more careful research using matched populations is needed, preliminary figures suggest that new HMOs perform much like mature HMOs;[73] this implies that HMOs are apparently a structural solution independent of the particular physicians and managers involved. Third, virtually all existing prepaid medical care foundations have formed in response to competition from HMOs, implying that competition by alternative systems can impact the behavior of traditional providers. If these findings are generalizable—and it seems highly probably that they are[74]—this model should effectively reduce cost escalation, maintain effectiveness, and improve efficiency if alternative systems become sufficiently numerous. Indeed if efficient alternative systems become sufficiently numerous, it can be argued that greater savings become possible because they will begin to affect the price of inputs. Present savings in alternative systems are achieved by controlling the use and mix of resources, but the price of resources—the price of a surgeon, for example—is determined by the larger traditional system. If alternative systems become numerous enough to reduce the demand for high style resources, the price of such resources should fall.

Financial protection and equity should be improved in a pluralistic medical care system of competing, comprehensive alternative and traditional provider plans and universal coverage. Perhaps the greatest concern is that the incentives for economy may lead prepaid medical care organizations to underserve members to the point of jeopardizing health. It should be noted that peer review (inherent in organized medical care systems) and consumer choice act as incentives to maintain quality, and that the meager research on quality in mature HMOs does not substantiate this charge.[75] But the troubles with the new directly prepaid Medicaid plans in California (which are not strictly HMOs because the consumer market is limited to Medicaid recipients) suggest some alternative organizations may try to underserve.[76] Although even there the market seems to be working—Medicaid recipients by disenrolling seem to be shaking out the bad actors rather faster than the state has been able to disqualify them—some form of enabling regulation to prevent bad actors from getting into the business seems desirable, as well as on-going quality assurance controls. (Parenthetically, we wish there were equal concern that fee-for-service providers may be overserving to the point of jeopardizing health. The omission of necessary services appears no less dangerous than the over-provision of unnecessary services.[77] The same small minority of lax professionals who would presumably deliberately underserve in new alternative systems are with equal probability now overserving in the present system. Quality assurance needs attention right now in both systems, and the means to do it are within reach if we have the will.)[78]

Prospects for the Medical Care System. Under this model the private medical care system would be preserved but significantly restructured. At least half of medical professionals would be providing service through more or less integrated prepaid medical care organizations. Probably the majority of these would be hospital-based multispecialty group practice situations, since they are likely to be more efficient and attract more consumers. The majority would also be provider sponsored, since this is likely to appeal most to providers. Quality assurance regulation is also likely to be present in both the traditional and alternative systems.

Prospects for Implementation. Like MRI, this model is a most promising option with severe difficulties in implementation. In its favor, this model can be incrementally approached (see Section II constraints 1 and 2). The government can try to stimulate alternative systems by removing existing market, legal, administrative and reimbursement barriers to their development in private and public benefit programs.[79] Under such a "fair market" climate, efficient alternative systems would be expected to compete well and grow. Some effort is being made in this direction now.[80]

But the creation of alternative systems requires private initiative, particularly by physicians (pressure from large group buyers would also help). But physicians are quite comfortable in the present system, and have little motivation to change. Hence they are content with resisting change rather than proposing credible change strategies of their own. Alternative systems also must win acceptance from consumers (especially large group buyers); but there is little public understanding of them presently, and in an uncertain economy comprehensive coverage is hard to sell.

Alternative systems also face difficulties in that public utility regulation largely ignores the fact that their structures and incentives, and therefore their performances and their needs, are different from traditional providers. Thus alternative systems find themselves regulated for the sins of others. This not only destroys any incentive for professionals to enter alternative systems to escape cost controls in the traditional fee-for-service system, it can directly inhibit alternative systems. As just one example, HMOs use half as many beds per capita as the national average, yet they are all subject to Certificate of Need bed controls. They must go through the lengthy, uncertain application process just the same as the worst offending traditional hospital. Not only may they find themselves without beds for a growing enrollment, they may find the bed control agency captured by their traditional system competition and used to keep them from even getting into the market.[81] Thus present public utility controls, especially market entry controls, are at best a hindrance and at worst a danger to alternative systems.

These inhibiting factors combine to suggest that without greater understanding by both public and private decision-makers, there will be too few alternative delivery systems in the next few years for private restructuring to constitute a major force in a cost containment strategy, even though it would probably work.

Model 5. The Public Utility Allocation Model (Alias the British Model). The essential feature defining this model is that it places a publicly specified "lid" on the total health care budget. That is, the government decides in advance how much shall be spent each year for health care, and has some mechanism to allocate this amount, and no more, to the medical care system. A number of variants are possible depending on the allocation mechanism, ranging from a national health service[82] (somewhat analogous to the education system) in which all providers are employed by the government, to a tight public utility arrangement in which all private inputs—manpower, facilities and money—are to some degree controlled by the government. Common to all these variants will be a division of the country into health care districts headed by a district health care board which allocates resources to district providers from a fixed district budget. People in the district are entitled to comprehensive health care from providers in the district. There may be nominal cost-sharing by patients, but the majority of provider payments comes from the district board. Private third parties, if present, serve only as intermediaries.

Prospects for Cost Containment. Both analysis and experience suggest this model might contain costs. The point of the analysis is that unless the budget is fixed in advance, public utility controls are unlikely to work well. Conversely, unless there are quite strong public utility controls on inputs, it will be difficult to keep within the fixed budget. With both a fixed budget and controls, cost containment is likely to be successful.

The reasoning is as follows. In Model 2 it was shown that process controls (e.g., controls on individual services) are unlikely to work well. A far less demanding way to control the volume of procedures is to limit the number of professionals performing them. A less demanding way to control style is to limit the number of specialists and the number of facilities and technological equipment available. On the other hand, what these limits should be is a matter of medical as well as economic judgment. How is the district board to limit the demands of the medical care system for more manpower, facilities, and equipment, when all such demands will be defended as improvements in health care? The only response government can finally make is that funds are limited. The government will therefore have to use its limited funds as an incentive and control on providers by fixing the district health care budget. When providers recognize that the demands of one provider for more means that the others get less, there will be a powerful incentive for all providers to agree on a defensible set of priorities and a method of allocating resources. There will also have to be strong controls so that providers can not individually ignore the priorities and wangle more resources than agreed on. Given a fixed budget, providers themselves are likely to help the district board make the controls work, so the controls are likely to succeed.

Two kinds of evidence suggest that this model will contain costs: the experience of England, and of HMOs. The British use an allocated fixed budget, and have had the least cost escalation of all the western nations. This is to be contrasted with Canada, which has a multitude of public utility controls but an open-ended budget based on reimbursement of whatever is done. In 1971 Canada spent an estimated 7.1 percent of its GNP for health care[83] and its annual increase in expenditures averaged an estimated 12 percent over the previous decade.[84] The comparable figures for England were 5.3 percent of a much smaller GNP in 1973 and 9.2 percent average annual expenditure increases. This evidence suggests not only that a fixed allocated budget can contain costs, but that without it public utility controls do not work well. While complaints are often voiced about the British system, such complaints seem due more to the fact that England is not a rich country than to the organization of its medical care system; if it spent as much per capita as the U.S., these complaints would likely diminish. The point is that they have control. If they stand in long queues for elective hospital care, it is because they have decided to spend the money for other national priorities. They can decide and the United States presently cannot. With their health statistics equal to ours and their expenditures far less, it appears that their system, whatever its short-comings, has given them a tremendous bang for the pound.

A less direct kind of evidence comes from HMOs. In effect, HMOs are privately operated mini-Englands with consumer choice. Each HMO works under a fixed budget (although specified by the market rather than the government) and allocates its resources according to priorities. Again the results show cost containment and a bigger bang for the buck (see references under Model 4).

This model provides excellent financial protection. Further, if district budgets are apportioned on a per capita basis, equity should be reasonably good. There will always be a tendency of the well-off to seek private services at a standard higher than the public system supports, possibly a more troublesome problem in the United States than England because of the larger number of high incomes. Nevertheless, government has means to discourage this practice if there is social consensus that its prevalence threatens the basic equity of the majority. The school system provides one analogy of how this equity issue might work out.

There are two other concerns about this model: efficiency and responsiveness to consumers. Unlike the previous consumer market oriented models, which emphasize installing efficient, responsive market mechanisms which then determine overall resource use on the basis of consumer preferences, this model fixes overall resource use directly and has no automatic internal incentives to maximize efficiency and responsiveness. The model makes the implicit value assumption or pragmatic judgment that national health care goals will be better achieved by expert direction than individual consumer decisions. Efficient allocation and use of resources must therefore arise from a political and administrative decision-making apparatus, and there is neither a market nor any a priori "right" rules to guide these decisions. Two kinds of efficiency considerations figure in such decisions: are we devoting the right amount of resources to health care *vis à vis* other health and non-health priorities (e.g., what should the "lid" be); and are we getting maximum health and consumer satisfaction from these resources (e.g., are we using our given health care resources efficiently)? The difficulty and ambiguity of these decisions can be exemplified by analogies from experience. For example, are we overfinancing or underfinancing our court system; is the court system dispensing maximum and speedy justice with the resource it has? Health care resource questions will not be much easier.

The gross decisions, such as the overall "lid" itself, may be the most satisfactory, but there may be increased problems as the decisions work down to detailed medical activities and areas. Even on the gross decisions there is the well-known vulnerability of politicians to capitulate to determined, well-organized interest groups, which providers certainly are and will become more so under this model. (England's continued parsimony—underfinancing?—in health care may be more the result of its poverty than the resoluteness of its politicians in the face of provider demands.) As decisions come down to the detailed level and require increasing medical input, the vulnerability of the system to run more for the providers than for the consumers increases. Similarly with responsiveness, while the consumer will have at least some choice of provider he will have little choice of system. The large bureaucracy entailed then implies a fair danger of rigidity and impersonality. (The political implications of the large new bureaucracy required have been treated by Flash.)[85] As decisions and actions descend to the detailed level the spirit may tend more toward "we're working for Uncle Sam who has lots of bucks" than "we're in a tough competition for consumers."

Nevertheless the experience of England shows that it is possible to arrive at a system with which most consumers and providers are reasonably satisfied on the whole if not in every detail. If we establish good feedback mechanisms on patient outcomes and consumer satisfaction, and if we make district boards responsive to consumers, we can perhaps minimize problems with efficiency and responsiveness. Making allowances for the size, traditions, and wealth of the United States compared with England, we should be able to achieve reasonable cost control, equity, efficiency and responsiveness with this model. Our school system provides perhaps the best analogy of what to expect.

Prospects for the Medical Care System. Again, careful analogies drawn from the school system, making allowances that providers will likely be politically stronger than teachers, may offer the best foresight into this model. Thus providers will probably not make their own opportunities so much as be presented them by the district boards. The district boards in negotiation with providers will likely determine the numbers and location of positions open in each specialty, and the size and type of service to be offered at each facility. Professionals will be much more bound by the actions of their peers, and professional "unions" or their equivalents are likely to appear to bargain with the boards. Innovations will likely have to come through consensus rather than individual action, and meet the approval of established providers.

Prospects for Implementation. The prospects for implementing this proposal all at once are very slim, as experience with the Kennedy-Corman bill, a fixed budget public approach, indicates. The degree of public control of the medical care system required to make this model work is unprecedented in this country. It will have to be incrementally approached, and each step is likely to be strenuously resisted by providers and probably by insurors. Moreover, if consumers are given no cost-share under this model, only government will be interested in cost containment; government will then muster little public support to implement successively stronger controls. Since cost-sharing is extremely difficult to restore once it has been removed,[86] government should not be too generous at first. It can then trade reduced cost-sharing for public support or more stringent controls. In sum, it is likely that this model might work, but the strength of the controls needed suggest the nation will take a long time getting there if it tries to go this way. However, the possibility to incrementally implement the model greatly improves its eventual political prospects. The danger is that the nation may try to approach this model through Model 2 (piecemeal public utility controls) first. Model 6, presented next, may offer the more advantageous approach.

Model 6. The Public Utility Hospital Model. This model is the least articulated of the four that might work. It starts with the observation that the most substantial and rapidly inflating portion of the personal health care dollar goes for hospital care, presently about 45 percent of personal health care expenditures.[87] Comparatively, the amount going to physician services (21 percent), and especially just to inpatient physician services (an estimated 9 percent), is small relative to the hospital expense induced by physicians' activity. Moreover, the number of hospitals (less than 7000) seems far more manageable than the number of practicing physicians (almost 300,000), and physicians seem to have the professional and political power to maintain their incomes in all western countries no matter what their medical system. This suggests that controlling the physician portion of the health care dollar may be very difficult. On the other hand it may be possible to contain the more substantial induced hospital costs that physicians cause by concentrating public utility controls mainly on the hospitals rather than on the entire system as in the previous model.

Under the impetus of Medicare, the Cost of Living Council, and some of the states, considerable work on hospital reimbursement and regulation has been initiated.[88] But little work has been published which looks down the road to coherent models of where such regulation might or should lead. Somers[89] has conceptually pioneered a model of the hospital as the integrating structure for the medical care system, but so far analysts have given little attention to the incentives and controls to make this structure perform any differently than the present system. The following analysis offers some considerations as to the necessary structure and incentive changes that may be required before such a public utility hospital model might realistically be expected to work.

The analysis starts with the basic structure and incentive assumptions of Section III.A, to which we now add two additional incentive assumptions particularly relevant to hospitals. The first is that *hospitals are dependent on physicians for patients, and therefore compete for physicians rather than for patients directly*. Financial viability, and the stability afforded by financial growth, is a basic incentive of most organizations. For hospitals, revenues come primarily from patient care. The hospital is dependent on its medical staff for both patients and the supervision of care. But the physician medical staff is actually independent of the hospital. Thus hospitals appear to basically compete for doctors, and can be expected to do whatever is necessary to attract them. If the physician wants a bed, the hospital will do its best to have one available; if the physician wants to do cobalt therapy, the hospital will try to have a unit for him.

The second assumption is that *there are additional strong incentives for hospitals to increase bed capacity and the style of services offered.*[90] Prestige and peer reputation are powerful incentives to hospital administrators and boards. Prestige and reputation apparently accrue from size of the hospital, reputation of the medical staff, and the elaborateness of services offered. Hospitals appear to compete with each other over all these aspects. Additionally, administrators find building their hospital program professionally rewarding, and size can add financial stability if it can be financed. The community, represented by the boards, tends to want high quality services, all immediately available near home, and is less aware of costs, which are passed on to insurers. In the absence of patient outcome monitoring, all these incentives are reinforced by the tendency of physicians, hospitals, and the public to equate quality with high style. With these additional assumptions, a number of inferences can be drawn concerning present and future hospital behavior:

1. *Hospitals will tend to overbuild and overuse bed capacity and specialized service units.* The above incentives on hospitals all point toward overbuilding in their efforts to cater to physicians and increase financial strength and prestige. The costs will be passed on to third parties (assumption 4, Section III.A). (Evidence shows this is already the case, see III.B.2). Demand-based planning as opposed to population-based planning, used by Hill-Burton and most states will aggravate this overbuilding and overuse of beds.

2. *The provision of ambulatory facilities and ambulatory health insurance benefits will likely add to, rather than substitute for, hospital services under the present medical care system.* Both physicians and hospitals have powerful incentives to increase hospitalization, and few incentives not to. In the presence of excess capacity, hospitals are likely to move strongly into outpatient care as a source rather than a substitute for inpatient admissions. (Existing evidence is consistent with both points, showing little substitution under ambulatory benefits[91] and an increasing growth of hospital outpatient units.)[92]

3. *In the presence of simultaneous excess capacity and growing government cost control pressure, hospitals are likely (a) to accept regulation which limits competition (Certificate of Need is an example) and (b) to seek strength through bigness via affiliations and multi-hospital firms.* As government tries to slow the growth of the medical care pie, hospitals recognize that if any one of them tries to expand too rapidly it may mean a smaller slice for the others, as well as increased pressure on all. Regulation of new investments has frequently been accepted by producers in such situations[93] as the best way to keep out new competitors and force existing producers to respect the present division of the market. On the other hand, the growth of larger and fewer third parties, in particular the government, should also lead hospitals to start affiliating and merging into larger multi-hospital firms to gain greater financial strength, market rationalization and political counter-muscle.[94] Since strength rather than efficiency may be the more powerful motive—economies of scale at large hospital and multi-hospital sizes are unproven and may be outweighed by diseconomies[95] — such alliances may result in hospitals growing to uneconomic sizes if the costs can be passed on to third parties. (Certificate of Need laws are present in two-thirds of the states[96] and are required under the new federal planning law, PL 93-641. Cooperative ventures and multi-hospital affiliations are in their infancy but seem to be spreading.)[97]

4. *Weak third party payers, rather than cost reimbursement appears responsible for the cost pass-through to third parties. Incentive-reimbursement of fee-for-service hospitals is unlikely to change things unless all such hospitals and all third parties are required to participate.* It makes little difference whether hospitals are reimbursed for costs or for charges if the third party is too weakly positioned (III.A.4) to control the rise in either.[98] Voluntary incentive reimbursement and rate review schemes are likely to fail in the presence of competing hospitals, since no hospital will intentionally jeopardize its financial stability and ability to compete for physicians. If the reimbursement scheme is not mandatory, the hospitals will use their latitude to concentrate on elaborate service to fewer patients, to refuse subscribers of unfavorable third parties (including Medicare and Medicaid beneficiaries) or to pass costs to weaker third parties,

Any public utility regulation of hospitals is unlikely to succeed unless it can overcome the powerful structure and incentive pressures above. The arguments advanced under Model 2 and Model 5 seem equally convincing here: successful direct regulation of the quantity and style of individual hospital services appears unfeasible, and regulation of inputs also seems unlikely to work in the absence of a fixed total budget. Thus a public authority or board with a fixed total budget for all hospital expenditures in its area will be assumed a minimum ingredient in any public utility hospital model. Second, this District Board must have sufficient powers to assure that the hospitals in its district do not exceed this budget, taking into account that the medical staff is a principle determinant of what hospitals do. In particular, it must be able to severely dampen or redirect the competition of hospitals for physician staff, and the demands of the physician staff for more elaborately equipped institutions. Thus it is highly probable that any effective public utility hospital model must give the Board at least some regulatory power over hospital medical staffs as well.

For discussion, one potentially effective model will be suggested here. There may be other effective models less stringent, but present evidence leaves doubt that controls a great deal less powerful will be effective. Thus this model may indicate the nature of what is involved to make the public utility hospital concept work:

1. *The nation would be divided into hospital districts.* In each district a Board would be established with control of all hospital payment dollars in its district, including both hospital services and inpatient physician services. If private insurers are retained, they will pay a stipulated capitation for each subscriber to the District Board (insurers thus function as intermediaries and bear no risk for hospital care). If private insurers are eliminated, the District Board would receive the capitation from whatever federal, state or local tax mechanism was established. All hospitals in the district would be paid directly by the Board.

In this way the third party effect is reduced to a single Board which, because it has only a fixed sum of capitation money, has an imperative incentive to control cost. From experience, this would appear to be the only incentive powerful enough to make the Board not yield to the intense pressures of its hospitals for more money. Clearly there must be checks on the Boards' arbitrarily raising the capitation amount; for example, the capitation could be stipulated by the federal, state or local government.

2. *The Board would have power to fix the budget, the size, the type of service offered, and the number of medical staff positions in each specialty in all hospitals in the district.* The Board would annually negotiate each of these items with each hospital, subject of course to the Board not exceeding its own budget. Each hospital would have to cover its service costs and pay its medical staff for inpatient services from its annual budget, but could do so in any manner it desired. If a hospital is unable to stay within its budget or maintain acceptable quality, the Board shall have the power to reorganize that hospital's management. These controls set severe limits on the hospital's ability to compete for doctors, services and beds, and give hospital management a powerful incentive (threat of reorganization) to stay within its budget. In turn, the hospital is given much greater control over its medical staff, since it now decides how they shall be paid for inpatient services, and medical staff positions are limited. The medical staff will know that requests for elaborate equipment, convenient operating room hours, etc., will come out of the same budget from which they are paid, and can be expected to moderate their demands. The Board has general

control over the number and distribution of services performed in any hospital by virtue of controlling the numbers of specialty positions, service mix and size of the hospital. The Board can thus distribute hospital services and medical staffing throughout the community as it deems best. It can reward efficient hospitals by granting them additional resources, and penalize inefficient hospitals by taking them away. The Board may also choose to buy tertiary care from other districts rather than maintain its own. (Some federal or state control may be necessary to prevent districts in professionally attractive areas from augmenting their budget from such sales to the point where they monopolize specialty care. Physicians could be expected to hospitalize less since their fees for non-inpatient care would not be controlled in this model; presumably ambulatory care would be subject to stiff consumer cost-sharing for all but low income consumers, exerting a market control on ambulatory care fees.)

Prospects for Cost Control. In the absence of experience, it is of course conjecture that such powerful controls will be necessary before cost escalation and maldistribution are held to acceptable amounts. It may be possible and more desirable, for example, to use an incentive reimbursement scheme rather than negotiation to allocate the fixed budget. But even with such variants, given the strong incentives for hospitals and the failure of existing regulation to work well, good arguments can be made that without a fixed budget and at least some regulatory power over hospital budget, size, service mix, and especially medical staff, it will be possible for physicians and hospitals to get around the Board, causing costs to rise excessively. With these controls, it seems quite possible that the public utility hospital model could be successful. There will be the same concerns about efficiency and responsiveness as in the previous model. It may succumb to the usual problems of public utility regulation—less than optimal efficiency, protection of existing firms, administrative rigidity and impersonality, and inhibitions toward innovation—but cost should be contained and distribution should be reasonably equitable. Thus, should the nation elect this path, this analysis suggests one down-the-road look at where we may end up.

Prospects for Implementation. Although less sweeping than the previous model, the controls necessary for this model to work effectively are sufficiently strong that they face formidable political obstacles. On the other hand, this model appears to have the best eventual political chance of any of the four models above because it can be staged incrementally. (This does not mean this model is better or worse than the other models, only that proponents of other models will have to work harder to get there.)

The question is one of time, how long it will take before the necessary controls can be enacted and given sufficient clout to be effective. Before the District Boards can be given a fixed budget, there will have to be an NHI plan giving universal hospital benefits to all persons in this district. Thus the control most indispensable to the model must await the enactment of NHI. The remaining controls can be started on now. The first step would be to divide the country into districts and begin building an administrative structure in each that would eventually become the District Boards. The next steps would be to successively give these agencies more control over hospital size, reimbursement, service mix, quality, and eventually (and most politically difficult) hospital medical staffing. While it may be necessary for the controls to be initially very weak in order to get enactment, the strategy would be to set precedents and then tighten them with subsequent legislation. Presumably this strategy could proceed swiftly enough so that by the time NHI were enacted, the structure and necessary precedents would be sufficiently in place for NHI to simply supply the capstone. If it proceeds too slowly for this, NHI could prove very inflationary, but this very pressure might speed implementation of the model under NHI.

The nation appears well along the road on this agenda. At least some supporters of the new HSAs apparently envision them as the eventual District Boards.[99] Precedents for control of hospital size and service mix already exist in the federal planning law creating the HSAs. Precedent to shift PSRO regulation from the local medical societies to other organizations (the HSAs?) exists in the PSRO law should the medical societies falter. (Conflict of interest difficulties make it not improbable that many of them will falter.) Regulation of specialty positions has only been raised so far in medical education bills, and has so far been defeated; the issue seems unlikely to die, and will be back again. Certainly precedents in these areas will be over the solid opposition of organized medicine, but cost pressures are eroding their strength.

The ease of implementation of this model thus rests on incrementally building on previous regulation. At each point the regulation is minimally disruptive; the government, bearing uncontrollable Medicare and Medicaid costs, has a powerful incentive to act; and the people, paying ever higher prices and premiums, will support the action. As in the previous model, perhaps the greatest danger to this strategy would be the too rapid elimination of private insurance and consumer cost-sharing. Once people were not faced with the high cost of care, they might be less likely to support firm government action.

V. Where Are We Headed: Some Conclusions

Perhaps the general conclusions to be drawn from the above analysis is that the structure and incentives producing the problems in our present medical care system are very strong and deep-rooted, and that adequate strategies to alter or counteract these incentives require substantial change that will be politically difficult to achieve. Of the four models examined that might work, our analysis has come up with the following suggestions.

The Major Risk Insurance Model. This would make the least overt change in the medical care system, requiring stringent controls only in specialized secondary and tertiary care. However, benefits must be legislated away to implement the model. But the political tendency in this and other countries is to erode cost-sharing. Thus it seems politically very difficult to obtain the kind of cost-sharing MRI requires, and equally difficult to sustain it if we ever did.

The Alternative Delivery Systems Model. This would preserve a pluralistic private medical care system, but involves substantial restructuring from the present system. The restructuring could occur in an evolutionary, incremental way, but there are presently few signs of the necessary public or private initiative, or understanding, to bring it about on the scale needed to make it effective generally.

The Public Utility Model. This would involve the greatest public intervention into the medical care system, most likely requiring fixed total budgets and public control over at least hospital size, service mix, reimbursement and medical staffing before it would work well. Although such controls can be approached incrementally, and government is strongly motivated to contain cost, it seems improbable that this magnitude of public intervention can be politically countenanced in the next few years.

A second conclusion is that the models politically most easy to fall into—generous financing with few or inadequate controls on the existing medical care system (Models 1 and 2)—are the most likely to aggravate and even rigidify all our present health care difficulties. While cost and equity pressures will eventually force us to more successful models, it will simply be longer, harder and more expensive to work our way out, and we may not come out as well.

A third conclusion is that there seems no reason not to incrementally proceed on all the potentially successful fronts at once—cost-sharing, alternative delivery systems and other provider incentive mechanisms, and public utility regulation aiming toward an allocated budget approach—before we attempt NHI. Thereby we could develop experience and explore models combining all three cost containment methods. If feasible, an eventual model marrying both consumer market and public utility cost containment methods may be more effective and even more politically acceptable in the long run than the more single-minded approaches advanced in the models above. It would appear from the analysis that the health care dollar spectrum can be divided into regimes where each method might work most optimally: Cost-sharing would seem to work best on "first" dollars (e.g., ambulatory care) where health care is very elective and the consumer's decisions less difficult. Provider incentives might work best on first dollars and "middle" dollars (e.g., common hospital episodes) where consumer knowledge is inadequate and the volume of service makes regulation difficult. Public utility regulation might work best on middle and "last" dollars (e.g., specialized secondary and tertiary care) where financial protection precludes cost-sharing and heavy but equitable constraints on very expensive technology are needed.

On cost-sharing, at a minimum the Congress could use its insurance regulatory powers to make cost-sharing simple and understandable to the consumer, so that when he purchased health care he would know exactly what his liability would be. For example, every insurance policy could be required to have only one deductible, one coinsurance rate, one maximum limit, and no inside limits, which apply to all benefits covered in the policy and are clearly stated on the cover. This might be one part of a larger "Truth in Health Insurance" Act. (More ambitiously, the Congress might additionally consider mandating that every insurer offer a federally specified non-income related Major Risk Insurance policy (say, threshold $2000, coinsurance 50 percent) as a dual choice to all group policies currently sold. No insurer would be permitted legally to sell a supplemental policy to a holder of MRI. Any employee electing MRI would receive the dollar difference between the MRI premium and his present group benefits as tax free income. Since such benefits are now tax free, this would cost the country nothing, the individual would not be coerced, and bargained benefits would not be disturbed. It could then be determined whether consumers would choose MRI voluntarily. While cost-sharing might never be prevalent enough to contain costs by itself, it will help. And if there is no cost-sharing, government will find poor public support for its efforts to contain costs.

With respect to alternative delivery systems, Congress could make the HMO Act more flexible to encourage a greater variety of directly prepaid medical care organizations, improve the reimbursement formula for qualified alternative systems under Medicare and Medicaid, and remove inappropriate regulation, such as Certificate of Need, from qualified alternative systems. Even if such alternative systems never become prevalent enough to contain all medical care costs by themselves, they will help.

With respect to public utility regulation, the Congress through its legislative authority over insurance could give the HSAs power to set fee-for-service hospital reimbursement rates uniformly for all insurers in its area. This would convert the country into a massive set of nonvoluntary incentive reimbursement[100] experiments. Reimbursement authority is an appropriate precedent, should HSAs eventually control total district health care budgets. In the absence of fixed budgets, the Congress will have to devise an effective carrot or stick to motivate the HSAs to effectively exercise their authority—not an easy task. Even if the HSAs do not succeed in containing hospital costs without a fixed budget, reimbursement controls will at least set a precedent for the day when fixed area-wide budgets are possible.

In practice such a multi-model approach may be difficult to keep consistent. The greatest administrative effort will necessarily be devoted to public utility regulation of the fee-for-service system, which may tend to build a large constituency in the bureaucracy sympathetic to this approach, so that the other approaches are neglected. And in general, interest groups have found it easier to live with regulation than true competition.

A final consideration in where we may be headed is the political line-up itself. The Administration and three of the four congressional committees which handle health legislation are normally characterized as moderate to conservative. The recent passage of strong regulatory health legislation (PSRO, HSAs) in the public utility vein—especially at a time when conservatives are considering deregulation in other industries—may therefore come as a surprise, and requires some explanation.

One explanation may lie in the perceptions of the various contending forces. One group, primarily liberals, have long been convinced that change is necessary. They see health care as a merit good in which price and market competition have little place; government must step in strongly and guarantee equitable access. A second group are practical, action-minded non-idealogues who see problems in the programs for which they are responsible. They are looking for the fastest way to get on top of their programs, and regulation appears the most immediate way to move. The last group, the conservatives, are still fighting the battle between change and no change.[101] Consequently, the conservatives are not writing much legislation for the health care system, whereas the other two groups, although not always in step with each other, are constantly coming forward with regulation-oriented bills. But even the conservatives must face the problems, which do not go away, especially the cost escalation problem. Having no strategy of their own for the medical care system, they must use whatever legislation is on the table, which is regulation-oriented. Thus the regulation-oriented bills may pass or fail depending on the pressures of the moment, but they keep coming back. They are the only credible ideas managing to reach the legislative table.

Considering the time and difficulty consumer market-oriented approaches will have in mustering sufficient private initiative to actually begin bringing the problems under control, and that conservatives are still hung up on whether change is necessary, the public utility-oriented approaches seem more likely to prevail, that is, unless the conservatives have a rather quick change of heart and convince the non-idealogues that a reformed consumer market does have a place in the future medical care system. Perhaps the major question now is whether the regulation will be coherent and unified, or fragmented and inconsistent. This depends on whether all the proponents of regulation understand how powerful the regulation will likely have to be before it becomes effective, and whether they agree on where the system is headed down the road. Even so, acquiring the necessary control will take much time and effort despite the fact that it can be approached incrementally.

A final question is whether the American public understands and accepts the change that will be required in its medical care system. The difficulty of implementing any workable approach is likely to require reasonable public consensus. As demonstrated by the illustrative models presented here, Americans have very genuine options, representing very different values, methods and consequences. If the public is divided on what should be done and what the future medical care system should be, this may frustrate a rational approach.

Thus it is hoped that public understanding and consensus might be built by having public figures and the media hold up the different alternatives for the future medical care system to public scrutiny and debate. Should we enact a generous national health insurance plan with only inadequate, inconsistent controls instead of a rational strategy for the medical care system—be it market-oriented, utility-oriented, or both—the nation could take a fairly expensive bath.

Notes

Notes

Chapter 1
Health, Health Costs, and Public Policy

1. Victor Fuchs, *Who Shall Live? Health Economics and Social Choice.* (New York: Basic Books, 1974), p. 17.

2. René Dubos, *Mirage of Health: Utopias, Progress and Biological Change* (New York: Harper & Row, 1959), p. 2.

3. Seymour E. Harris, *The Economics of Health Care: Finance and Delivery* (Berkeley, Calif.: McCutchan Publishing Corporation, 1975), pp. 63-67.

4. Ibid.

5. Stephen Strickland, *Politics, Science and Dread Disease: A Short History of United States Medical Research Policy* (Cambridge, Mass: Harvard University Press, 1972), pp. 210-232.

6. See Harry Schwartz, "On Medical Progress," *New York Times,* April 13, 1976. Also see Jane E. Brody, "Popular New X-Ray Unit Could Raise Cost of Care," *New York Times,* May 8, 1976; and Howard M. Hiatt, MD, "Too Much Medical Technology?" *The Wall Street Journal,* June 24, 1976.

7. See Richard Spark, MD, "The Case Against Regular Physicals," *New York Times Magazine,* July 25, 1975, pp. 10-11, 38-41.

8. Lester Breslow, "Preventive Medical Services in National Health Policy," paper presented at the 103rd Annual Meeting of the American Public Health Association, Chicago, Illinois, November 1975.

9. Quoted in Rick J. Carlson, *The End of Medicine* (New York: John Wiley & Sons, 1975), p. 192.

10. Leon S. White, "Sounding Board: How to Improve the Public's Health," *The New England Journal of Medicine,* Vol. 293, No. 15, October 9, 1975, pp. 773-774.

11. Daniel P. Moynihan, *Forward to Federal Health Spending 1969-74* (Washington: Center for Health Policy Studies, National Planning Association, 1974), p. iii.

12. Marjorie Smith Mueller and Robert M. Gibson, "National Health Expenditures, Fiscal Year 1975," *Social Security Bulletin,* Vol. 39, No. 2, February 1976, pp. 3-20.

13. Congressional Budget Office, "Budget options for fiscal year 1977: A Report to the Senate and House Committees on the Budget (Washington: U.S. Government Printing Office, March 15, 1976), pp. 151-168.

14. Executive Office of the President, Council on Wage and Price Stability, Staff Report, "The Problem of Rising Health Care Costs," April 1976.

15. Ibid.

16. U.S. Department of Health, Education and Welfare, National Center for Health Statistics, "Health Resource Statistics, 1974."

17. Ibid.

18. Ibid.

19. U.S. Department of Health, Education and Welfare, "Medical Care Expenditures, Prices and Costs: Background Book," September 1975, p. 42.

20. See Robert M. Ball, in Joseph G. Perpich, ed., *Implications of Guaranteeing Medical Care* (Washington: National Academy of Sciences, 1976), p. 39.

21. Marjorie Smith Mueller and Paula A. Piro, "Private Health Insurance in 1974: A Review of Coverage, Enrollment and Financial Experience," *Social Security Bulletin*, Vol. 39, No. 3, March 1976, pp. 3-20.

22. Ibid.

23. Victor Fuchs, "The Basic Forces Influencing Costs of Medical Care," in Fuchs, ed., *Essays in the Economics of Health and Medical Care* (New York: National Bureau of Economic Research, 1972), pp. 41-42. Also see his essays, "The Contribution of Health Service to the American Economy," pp. 3-39 and "The Growing Demand for Medical Care," pp. 61-69 in the same volume.

24. H.E. Frech III, "Regulatory Reform: The Case of the Medical Care Industry," in W.S. Moore, ed., *Regulatory Reforms: Highlights of a Conference on Government Regulation* (Washington: American Enterprise Institute for Public Policy Research, 1976), p. 16.

25. Ibid.

26. See, for example, F.J. Ingelfinger, "Deprofessionalizing the Profession," *The New England Journal of Medicine*, Vol., No. February 5, 1976, p. 334.

27. Robert R. Alford, *Health Care Politics: Ideological and Interest Group Barriers to Reform* (Chicago: The University of Chicago Press, 1975).

28. Ibid.

29. Ibid., p. 6.

30. Ibid., p. 6.

31. See Arnold Weber, "The Continuing Courtship: Wage-Price Policy Through Five Administrations," in Crawford D. Goodwin, ed., *Exhortation and Controls: The Search for a Wage-Price Policy 1945-1971* (Washington: Brookings, 1975), pp. 353-385.

32. See chapter 4.

33. See, for example, Jonathan Spevak, "Prescription Flap: Federal Plan to Control Prices on Drugs in Medicare, Medicaid Sets off a Dispute," *The Wall Street Journal*, April 27, 1976, p. 40.

34. Fuchs, *Who Shall Live?*, p. 5.

35. Ibid., p. 7.

36. Ibid.

37. See chapter 8, p. 223.

Chapter 2
The Social Security Administration and Medicare:
A Strategy of Implementation

1. 42 USC 1395 x (c) and (k).

2. See 42 USC 1395 bb.

3. See *The Character and Implications of SSA's Administration of* Medicare, Denver: Spectrum Research, Inc., 1975, Chapter II; based on HIBAC minutes, I: 2, November 13, 1965, pp. 14–16; "Conditions for Participation for Hospitals," draft, December 16, 1965, HIBAC Agenda Book, December 17–19, 1965; 20 C.F.R. 405. 1003–1011; HIBAC minutes, III: December 19, 1965.

4. "The Role of Fiscal Intermediaries in Claims Review," staff memorandum for HIBAC, in HIBAC Agenda Book, June 3-4, 1967: HIBAC minutes, XVI: 2, June 4, 1967, pp. 21-22; Sylvia Law, *Blue Cross; What Went Wrong,* New Haven, Yale University Press, 1974, p. 122 and notes 672 and 673.

5. See Law, *Blue Cross.*

6. Interviews with officials in SSA and PHS; "Summary of Program Review Findings and State Agency Recommendations," and "Selected State Reports," in HIBAC, Task Force on Hospital and Extended Care Services, September-December 1968; "Need for Timely Action in Resolving Problems Affecting the Eligibility of Hospitals Under the Medicare Program," B-164031 (4) SSA, HEW, by the Comptroller General of the U.S., December 27, 1968.

7. HIBAC's First Annual Report, p. 10.

8. Interviews with SSA and PHS officials.

9. Personal interviews with responsible officials.

10. See "Reimbursement Guidelines for Medicare," Hearings before the Committee on Finance, U.S. Senate, 89: 2, May 25, 1966.

11. See, for example, Martin S. Feldstein, *The Rising Cost of Hospital Care,* published for the National Center for Health Services Research and Development, U.S. Department of Health, Education and Welfare, Washington, D.C.: Information Resources Press, 1971.

12. Account based on personal interviews with senior Medicare officials.

13. Personal interview with BHI official.

14. See "1967 Social Security Recommendations, Summary of Major Proposals," p. 3, in HIBAC Agenda Book, March 4, 1967; and "President's

Proposals for Revisions in the Social Security System," Hearings before Committee on Ways and Means on HR 5710, House of Representatives, 90:1, p. 42 ff.

15. Irwin Wolkstein, in U.S. Government, HEW, SSA, ORS, "Reimbursement Incentives for Hospital and Medical Care; Objectives and Alternatives," Research Report No. 26, Washington, D.C.: U.S. Government Printing Office, 1968, p. 14.

16. Personal interviews with responsible officials and congressional participants.

17. "Status of Program Experimentation in the Bureau of Health Insurance," staff memorandum for HIBAC, November 28, 1972, p. 1.

18. Official quoted by John K. Iglehart, in "Health Report/Prepaid Group Practice Emerges as likely Federal Approach to Health Care," *National Journal,* 3:28 (July 10, 1971), p. 1449.

19. See "Medicare and Medicaid: Problems, Issues and Alternatives," Report of the staff to the Finance Committee, U.S. Senate, Committee Print, 91st Cong., 1st session, February 9, 1970; and "Medicare and Medicaid: Hearings," Part 1; Senate Finance Committee, 91st Cong., 2nd session, 1970.

20. See "Medicare and Medicaid: Hearings," pp. 6-7.

21. Interviews with BHI officials; HIBAC documents, in particular, "Background Material for the Council's Intended Discussion of Medical Costs," Staff Memorandum for HIBAC, HIBAC Agenda Book, January 10-11, 1970.

22. Ibid.

23. Personal interviews with BHI officials.

24. Personal interviews with responsible officials.

25. See footnote j, p. 42.

26. See "Administration of Federal Health Benefit Programs," Hearings before the Subcommittee of the Committee on Government Operations, House of Representatives, 91/1, part 1, pp. 42-45.

27. "Social Security Amendments of 1970," Report of the Committee on Finance, U.S. Senate, to Accompany HR 17550, Senate Report 91-1431, December 11, 1970, p. 179; Interviews with participants; and HIBAC minutes, clearance draft, XXXVII:2, March 27, 1971, p. 15; HIBAC Agenda Book, April 23-24, 1971.

28. Interviews with BHI officials; "Social Security Amendments of 1970," Ways and Means Report on HR 17750, May 14, 1970, pp. 39-45; "Clarifying the Meaning of Reasonable Cost Under Title XVIII, in HIBAC Agenda book, March 21-22, 1970.

29. "Meeting on HMO Policy Issues, Baltimore, Maryland, September 17, 1971," p. 1, included in "HMO Policy Issues," staff memorandum for HIBAC, HIBAC Agenda Book, October 15-16, 1971.

30. Personal interviews with BHI officials.

31. Ibid; and *Character and Implications,* Chapter VII.

32. Interviews with participants.

33. See Theodore R. Marmor, Donald A. Wittman, and Thomas C. Heagy, "Politics, Public Policy and Medical Inflation," in *Health: A Victim or Cause of Inflation,* Michael Zubcoff, ed., New York: Milbank Memorial Fund, 1975, pp. 19-21.

34. Ibid.

Chapter 3
**Implementation of the End-Stage Renal Disease Program:
A Mixed Pattern of Subsidizing and Regulating the
Delivery of Medical Services**

1. Comptroller General of the United States, *Treatment of Chronic Kidney Failure: Dialysis, Transplant, Costs, and the Need for More Vigorous Efforts (Department of Health, Education, and Welfare),* Washington, D.C., U.S. General Accounting Office, June 24, 1975, pp. 38-39.

2. Ibid., pp. 43-44.

3. U.S. House of Representatives, Committee on Ways and Means, *Background Information on Kidney Disease Benefits Under Medicare,* Committee Print, 94th Congress, 1st Session, June 24, 1975, p. 3. Hereafter, Ways and Means, *Background Information.*

4. Ibid.

5. Public Law 92-603, "Social Security Amendments of 1972," 92nd Congress, October 30, 1972, pp. 135-136.

6. Ways and Means, *Background Information,* p. 15.

7. Ibid., p. 6.

8. See "Payment for Services in Connection with Kidney Transplant and Renal Dialysis Provided to Entitled Beneficiaries," *Federal Register,* Vol. 38, No. 125, June 29, 1971, pp. 17210-17212 (hereafter, Interim Regulations).

9. U.S. Congress, *Congressional Record—Senate,* 92nd Congress, 2nd Session, September 30, 1975, pp. S16396-16402.

10. See "Kidney Disease Treatment Program of Medicare," remarks by Ronald M. Klar, M.D., special assistant for health policy development, Department of Health, Education, and Welfare, to the Annual Meeting of the National Kidney Foundation, Washington, D.C., November 16, 1973.

11. See remarks by Charles C. Edwards, M.D., assistant secretary for health, Department of Health, Education, and Welfare, at a press briefing, June 26, 1973, announcing the Interim Regulations, p. 3.

12. Interim Regulations, pp.17210-17211.

13. Statement later published as: "Facilities Providing Treatment for End-Stage Renal Disease; Interim Period Qualification and Exception Criteria," *Federal Register,* Vol. 39, No. 194, October 4, 1974, pp. 35811-35819.

14. Sylvester Berki, *Hospital Economics,* (Lexington, Mass., Lexington Books, D.C. Heath and Company, 1972, p. 185).

15. U.S. Department of Health, Education, and Welfare, Social Security Administration, Part A Intermediary Letter No. 73-25, Part B Intermediary Letter No. 73-22, "Processing and Payment of Claims for Renal Dialysis and Transplant Services Performed for Eligible Medicare Beneficiaries after June 30, 1973," July 1973.

16. Memorandum, from the director, Office of Health Financing Policy Development, to the assistant secretary for health, "Kidney Disease Treatment Program of Medicare—Reimbursement Policy Issues—*ACTION,*" December 19, 1973, revised January 4, 1975, revised February 12, 1974, p. 5.

17. Interim Regulations, p. 17212.

18. Ibid.

19. Part A Intermediary Letter No. 73-25, Part B Intermediary Letter 73-22, p. 19.

20. U.S. Department of Health, Education, and Welfare, Social Security Administration, Part A Intermediary Letter No. 74-24, "Payment for Dialysis Treatments Provided During a Hospital Inpatient Stay," July 1974.

21. See U.S. Department of Health, Education, and Welfare, Press Release, April 17, 1974, Remarks by Charles C. Edwards, M.D., assistant secretary for health, New York City, April 17, 1974, and "Final Policies: P.L. 92-603, Section 299I, End-Stage Renal Disease Program of Medicare," April 1974.

22. U.S. Department of Health, Education, and Welfare, Social Security Administration, Part A Intermediary Letter No. 74-20, Part B Intermediary Letter No. 74-20, "Alternative Reimbursement Method of Monthly Payments to Physicians for Services Rendered to Patients on Maintenance Dialysis," June 1974, p. 3.

23. "Final Policies," p. 8.

24. Ibid., pp. 39-50.

25. See S. 1492, Introduced in the Senate of the United States, April 21, 1975, by Senator Russell B. Long. See also U.S. House of Representatives, Committee on Ways and Means, *Background Information on Kidney Disease Benefits Under Medicare,* Committee Print, 94th Congress, 1st Session, June 24, 1975; *Medicare's Kidney Disease Benefits Program,* Hearings, 94th Congress, 1st Session, June 24, and July 30, 1975; and *Report on Administration by the Social Security Administration of the End-Stage Renal Disease Program Established by Public Law 92-603 and On Social Security Medicare Research Studies,* Committee Print, 94th Congress, 1st Session, October 22, 1975.

Chapter 4
Drug-Cost Control: The Road to Maximum
Allowable-Cost Regulations

1. Limitations on Payment or Reimbursement for Drugs, *Federal Register,* Vol. 40, No. 148, July 31, 1975, p. 32303.

2. Maximum Allowable Cost for Drugs, *Federal Register,* Vol. 40, No. 159, August 15, 1975, p. 34519.

3. U.S. Senate, Committee on the Judiciary, Subcommittee on Antitrust and Monopoly, *Administered Prices in the Drug Industry,* Washington, D.C.: U.S. Government Printing Office. See also Kefauver, Estes, *In a Few Hands: Monopoly Power in America,* (Baltimore: Penguin Books, 1965).

4. U.S. Senate, Select Committee on Small Business, Subcommittee on Monopoly, *Competitive Problems in the Drug Industry,* Washington, D.C.: U.S. Government Printing Office, 1967.

5. U.S. Department of Health, Education and Welfare, Office of the Secretary, Task Force on Prescription Drugs, *Final Report,* Washington, D.C.: U.S. Government Printing Office, 1969; also *The Drug Users,* 1968; *The Drug Makers and the Drug Distributors,* 1968; *Current American and Foreign Programs,* 1968; *Approaches to Drug Insurance Design,* 1969.

6. Silverman, Milton, and Philip R. Lee, *Pills, Profits, and Politics.* (Los Angeles: University of California Press, 1974, p. 35).

7. Ibid., p. 35.

8. HEW Task Force, *Final Report,* p. 31; *The Drug Makers and Drug Prescribers,* p. 23; and U.S. Senate, *Competitive Problems in the Drug Industry,* Part 20, pp. 7966-7994.

9. HEW Task Force, *Final Report,* p. 8.

10. Kefauver, Estes, *In a Few Hands,* pp. 77-78. Prior to the passage of this law only proof of safety was required.

11. Silverman and Lee, pp. 110-116.

12. Talley, Robert B., and Laventurier, Marc F., "Drug Utilization and Peer Review in San Joaquin," presented before the American Association Foundations for Medical Care, August 28, 1972.

13. G.R. Mundy, et al., "Current Medical Practice and the Food and Drug Administration," Journal of the American Medical Association, Vol. 229, No. 13, September 23, 1974, pp. 1744-1748.

14. Melmon, Kenneth L., "Preventable Drug Reactions: Causes and Cures," *New England Journal of Medicine,* June 17, 1971.

15. Maronde, Robert F., *Drug Utilization Review with On Line Computer Capability,* Social Security Administration, Office of Research and Statistics: DHEW Publication No. (SSA) 73-11853, Staff Paper No. 13.

16. California Department of Health News Release, June 23, 1975. See also Wisconsin Assembly Bill 1387.

17. U.S. Senate, Committee on Labor and Public Welfare, Subcommittee on Health, *Examination of the Pharmaceutical Industry,* Washington, D.C.: U.S. Government Printing Office. Testimony by Secretary Weinberger, December 19, 1973.

18. Maximum Allowable Cost for Drugs, *The Federal Register,* Vol. 39, No. 222, November 15, 1974.

19. *Federal Register,* Vol. 40, No. 148, July 31, 1975, p. 32285.

20. U.S. Congress, Office of Technology Assessment, *Drug Bioequivalence,* July 1974.

21. U.S. Senate, Select Committee on Small Business, Subcommittee on Small Business, *Competitive Problems in the Drug Industry,* Part 26, pp. 11656-11657.

22. *Federal Register,* Vol. 40, No. 148, July 31, 1975, p. 32285.

23. Limitations on Payment on Reimbursement for Drugs, *Federal Register,* Vol. 40, No. 148, July 31, 1975.

24. Ibid., p. 32303.

25. Maximum Allowable Cost for Drugs, *Federal Register,* Vol. 40, No. 159, August 15, 1975, p. 34514.

26. *American Medical Association vs. Caspar W. Weinberger,* U.S. District Court for the Northern District of Illinois, Eastern Division.

27. Speech by Senator Herman Talmadge before the National Association of Retail Druggists, February 25, 1976.

Chapter 5
Medical Politics and Medical Prices: The Relation between
Who Decides and How Much It Costs

1. See Harris S. Cohen, "Professional Licensure, Organizational Behavior, and the Public Interest," *Milbank Memorial Fund Quarterly,* 51 (Winter 1973) 73-88.

2. J.C. Record, "The Research Institute and the Pressure Group," in G. Sjoberg (ed.), *Ethics, Politics, and Social Research* (Cambridge, Mass: Schenkman, 1967), 43-46.

3. M. Friedman, *Capitalism and Freedom* (Chicago: University of Chicago Press, 1962), Chapter 9.

4. Eliot Freidson, *Profession of Medicine* (New York: Dodd, Mead, 1970).

5. *Hearings,* Committee on the Judiciary, Subcommittee on Antitrust and Monopoly, U.S. Senate, 93d Cong., 2d Sess., Parts 1 and 2, 1974.

6. *The Wall Street Journal,* December 24, 1975, p. 2; *New York Times,* February 27, 1976, p. 33.

7. *Washington Report on Medicine and Health,* 30, April 19, 1976, p. 2.

8. Speech to the Senate, July 1, 1970. Reprinted in *Background Material Relating to Professional Standards Review Organizations (PSRO's),* prepared by the staff of the Senate Committee on Finance, U.S. Government Printing Office, May 8, 1974, p. 47, including the PSRO section of the Committee's September 26, 1972 report, *Social Security Amendments of 1972,* prepared to accompany H.R. 1 of the 92nd Congress, 2nd Session (Senate Report No. 92-1230).

9. Ibid., p. 4.

10. *PSRO Program Manual,* Office of Professional Standards Review, Washington, D.C., 1974.

11. See, for example, "What 1,000 Family Doctors Think About the PSRO Situation," *Medical Times,* 102 (July 1974), 102-111; and "Blueprint for Control: No-knock Peer Review," *Modern Hospital,* 121, 1 (July 1973), 7-10.

12. *New York Times,* December 6, 1973, p. 1; see also December 3, 1973, p. 1 and December 4, 1973, p. 14.

13. *PSRO Letter* (published semimonthly by McGraw-Hill, Washington, D.C.), April 1, 1974.

14. C.E. Welch, "PSROs—Pros and Cons," *New England Journal of Medicine,* 290, June 6, 1974, 1319-1322.

15. Ibid.

16. *PSRO Letter,* July 15, 1974, p. 5

17. Ibid., p. 5. See also *New York Times,* June 30, 1974, IV, p. 9.

18. *Federal Register,* March 30, 1974, p. 13453.

19. W.B. Munier, acting director of HEW's Bureau of Quality Standards, in a letter to the *New York Times,* as quoted in *PSRO Letter,* March 1, 1976.

20. *PSRO Letter,* March 1, 1976 first reports from PSROs have been mixed. The time has been too short and the factors too complex to develop conclusive evidence.

21. Ibid. Although Congress patently viewed PSROs as a cost containment instrument, HEW under Secretary Mathews appears to be less cost conscious than it was under Secretary Weinberger.

22. Social Security Amendments of 1972, p. 260.

23. *American Hospital Medical Education Journal (AHMEJ),* Spring 1976, p. 11.

24. From personal conversations in March and April 1976.

25. *AHMEJ,* Ibid., p. 12.

26. See, for example, *Physicians for a Growing America,* Report of the Surgeon General's Consultant Group on Medical Education, U.S. Department of Health, Education, and Welfare (Washington: U.S. Government Printing Office, October 1959), often referred to as the Bane report.

27. Report of the National Advisory Commission on Health Manpower, Volumes I and II (Washington: U.S. Government Printing Office, November 1967).

28. The Health Manpower Act of 1968 (Public Law 90-490) and the Health Training Improvement Act of 1970 (Public Law 91-519).

29. *Higher Education and the Nation's Health: Policies for Medical and Dental Education* (New York: McGraw-Hill, 1970).

30. Report by the Committee on Interstate and Foreign Commerce, U.S. House of Representatives, 94th Congress, 1st Session, June 9, 1975 (Report No. 94-266, to accompany H.R. 5546, a health manpower bill). Also, report by the Committee on Labor and Public Welfare, U.S. Senate, 94th Congress, 2nd Session, May 14, 1976 (Report No. 94-266, to accompany S. 3239). Hereafter, references to Senate and House committees and reports are to the committees and volumes cited here, unless otherwise noted.

31. House Committee Report, p. 16.

32. Senate Committee Report, p. 34.

33. Ibid., pp. 36ff.

34. Ibid., p. 42.

35. Emergency Health Personnel Act Amendments, contained in Public Law 92-585.

36. House Committee Report, 21. (See views of committee members who opposed capitation replayment, beginning at p. 249).

37. Senate Report, p. 47.

38. Ibid., p. 201.

39. Senate Report, p. 202.

40. House Committee Report, p. 55.

41. *Hearings,* I, pp. 886-887 (see footnote o, p. 94).

Chapter 6
The Limits of Regulation: Implications of Alternative
Models for the Health Sector

1. Randall Ripley, "Introduction, The Politics of Public Policy," in Ripley, ed. *Public Policies and Their Politics* (New York: Norton, 1966), pp. vii-xvi.

2. Cf. Theodore J. Lowi, "Decision Making Vs. Policy Making: Toward an Antidote for Technocracy," XXX, *Public Administration Review* (May–June 1970), pp. 314–325.

3. Cf. George D. Greenberg, Jeffrey A. Miller, Lawrence B. Mohr, and Bruce C. Vladeck, "Developing Public Policy Theory: Perspectives From Empirical Research," *American Political Science Review,* December 1977 (forthcoming).

4. Cf. *Congressional Record,* February 18, 1976, p. H1134.

5. Majorie Smith Mueller and Robert M. Gibson, "National Health Expenditures, Fiscal Year 1975," 39, *Social Security Bulletin* (February 1976), p. 14.

6. Cf. Harris S. Cohen, "Professional Licensure, Organizational Behavior, and the Public Interest," 51, *The Milbank Memorial Fund Quarterly: Health and Society* (Winter 1973), pp. 73–88.

7. Victor R. Fuchs, *Who Shall Live?: Health, Economics, and Social Choice* (New York: Basic Books), 1974, pp. 82–83.

8. Ibid., p. 12.

9. Cf. Bruce C. Vladeck, "Why Non-Profits Go Broke," 42, *The Public Interest* (Winter 1976), pp. 86–101.

10. Cf. Louise B. Russell and Carol S. Burke, "Technological Diffusion in the Hospital Sector" (Washington: National Planning Association, October 1975).

11. Cf. Wallace J. Lovejoy, "The Impact of Competition Among Public Utilities: Gas Versus Electricity," in Harry M. Trebing, ed., *Essays on Public Utility Pricing and Regulation* (East Lansing, Mich.: Institute of Public Utilities, 1971), pp. 213–243.

12. Cf. Martin S. Feldstein, "Hospital Cost Inflation: A Study of Nonprofit Price Dynamics," 61, *American Economic Review* (December 1971), pp. 853–872; Maw Lin Lee, "A Conspicuous Production Theory of Hospital Behavior," 38, *Southern Economic Journal* (July 1971), pp. 48–55; Joseph P. Newhouse, "Toward a Theory of Nonprofit Institutions: An Economic Model of a Hospital," 60, *American Economic Review* (March 1970), pp. 64–74; Karen A. Davis, "Economic Theories of Behavior in Nonprofit, Private Hospitals," 24, *Economics and Business Bulletin* (Winter 1972), pp. 1–13; Vladeck, "Why Non-Profits Go Broke."

13. James W. McKie, "Regulation and the Free Market: The Problem of Boundaries," 1, *Bell Journal of Economics and Management Science* (Spring 1970), p. 9.

14. Marver F. Bernstein, *Regulating Business by Independent Commission* (Princeton, N.J.: Princeton University Press, 1955), pp. 217ff.

15. Cf. Theodore J. Lowi, *The End of Liberalism: Ideology, Policy, and the Crisis of Public Authority* (New York: Norton, 1969), pp. 86–87.

16. Cf. Herbert L. Packer, *The Limits of the Criminal Sanction* (Stanford, Calif.: Stanford University Press, 1968), pp. 354-363; Sanford H. Kadish, "Some Observations on the Use of Criminal Sanction in Enforcing Economic Regulations," 30, *University of Chicago Law Review* (Spring 1963), pp. 423-449; but contrast Harry V. Ball and Lawrence M. Friedman, "The Use of Criminal Sanctions in the Enforcement of Economic Legislation: A Sociological View," 17, *Stanford Law Review* (January 1965), pp. 197-223.

17. Cf. Albert W. Alschuler, "The Prosecutor's Role in Plea Bargaining," 36, *University of Chicago Law Review* (Autumn 1968), pp. 50-112.

18. Alvin W. Gouldner, *Patterns of Industrial Bureaucracy* (New York: The Free Press, 1954), pp. 174-176.

19. Cf. New York State Moreland Act Commission, *Regulating Nursing Home Care: The Paper Tigers,* Report Number 1 (New York: The Commission, October 1975); Patrick O'Donoghue, *Evidence About the Effects of Health Care Regulation: An Evaluation and Synthesis of Policy Relevant Research* (Denver, Colo.: Spectrum Research, Inc, 1974), Chapter VI.

20. Cf. Harold Cohen, "State Rate Regulation," in Institute of Medicine, National Academy of Sciences, *Controls on Health Care,* Proccedings of the Conference on Regulation in the Health Industry, January 7-9, 1974 (Washington: National Academy of Sciences, 1975), pp. 123-135.

21. Cf. Lewin and Associates, *An Analysis of State and Regional Health Regulation,* Vol. I: Report of the Study (Washington, D.C.: Lewin and Associates, February 1975), Chapter IV.

22. Cf. chapter 2.

23. Cf. chapter 4 for an example.

24. Cf. U.S. Congress, House of Representatives, Committee on Government Operations, *Department of Health, Education, and Welfare (Prevention and Detection of Fraud and Program Abuse),* Tenth Report, House Report No. 94-786, 94th Congress, 2nd Session (Washington: U.S. Government Printing Office, 1976).

25. Cf. U.S. Congress, Senate Special Committee on Aging, Subcommittee on Long-Term Care, *Nursing Home Care in the United States: Failure in Public Policy,* Supporting Paper No. 5, *The Continuing Chronicle of Nursing Home Fires,* Report No. 94-100, 94th Congress, 1st Session (Washington: U.S. Government Printing Office, 1975).

26. Gabriel Kolko, *Railroads and Regulation, 1877-1916* (Princeton: Princeton University Press, 1965); Mark Green and Ralph Nadar, "Economic Regulation vs. Competition: Uncle Sam and the Monopoly Man," 82, *Yale Law Journal* (April 1973), pp. 871-889.

27. Cf. Richard A. Posner, "Natural Monopoly and its Regulation," 21, *Stanford Law Review* (February 1969), p. 622; George J. Stigler, "The Process of Economic Regulation," 17, *Antitrust Bulletin* (Spring 1972), pp. 207-235.

28. Lowi, *End of Liberalism*, pp. 101ff.; Cf. Louis L. Jaffe, "The Effective Limits of the Administrative Process: A Reevaluation," 67, *Harvard Law Review* (May 1954), p. 1113.

29. Cf. Mancur Olson, *The Logic of Collective Action: Public Goods and the Theory of Groups* (Cambridge: Harvard University Press, 1965).

30. Cf. Walter Adams and William James Adams, "The Military-Industrial Complex: A Market Structure Analysis," 62, *American Economic Review Papers and Proceedings* (May 1972); Larry Paul Ellsworth, "Defense Procurement: Everyone Feeds at the Trough," in Mark J. Green, ed., *The Monopoly Makers: Ralph Nader's Study Group Report on Regulation and Competition* (New York: Grossman Publishers, 1973); Arthur E. Burns, "Profit Limitation: Regulated Industries and the Defense-Space Industries," 3, *Bell Journal of Economics and Management Science* (Spring 1972), pp. 3-25.

31. Rufus E. Miles, Jr., *The Department of Health, Education, and Welfare*, Praeger Library of U.S. Government Departments and Agencies (New York: Praeger, 1974), p. 179.

32. Cf. James S. Turner, Project Director, *The Chemical Feast: The Ralph Nader Study Group Report on Food Protection and the Food and Drug Administration* (New York: Grossman Publishers, 1970), p. 100.

33. Cf. Louis L. Jaffe, "The Illusion of the Ideal Administration," 86, *Harvard Law Review* (May 1973), pp. 1183-1199.

34. George W. Hilton, "The Basic Behavior of Regulatory Commissions," 62, *American Economic Review Papers and Proceedings* (May 1972), p. 48.

35. Cf. Roger G. Noll, *Reforming Regulation: An Evaluation of the Ash Council Proposals*, A Staff Paper, Studies on the Regulation of Economic Activities (Washington: The Brookings Institution, 1971), pp. 39-46; Warren J. Samuels, "Public Utilities and the Theory of Power," in Milton Russell, ed., *Perspectives in Public Regulation: Essays on Political Economy* (Carbondale, Ill.: Southern Illinois University Press, 1973), pp. 1-27.

36. Donald J. Newman, "Pleading Guilty for Considerations: A Study of Bargain Justice," 46, *Journal of Criminal Law, Criminology, and Police Science* (March-April 1956), pp. 780-790, is still authoritative.

37. Jerome H. Skolnick, "Social Control in the Adversary System," XI, *Journal of Conflict Resolution* (March 1967), pp. 52-63.

38. Cf. Albert O. Hirschman, *Exit, Voice, and Loyalty: Responses to Decline in Firms, Organizations, and States* (Cambridge: Harvard University Press, 1970), pp. 26-29.

39. Bernstein, *Regulating Business by Independent Commission*, pp. 74ff.; William L. Cary, *Politics and the Regulatory Agencies* (New York: McGraw-Hill, 1967), pp. 1-2 et. passim.; Samuel J. Huntington, "The Marasmus of the ICC: The Commission, the Railroads, and the Public Interest," in Peter Woll, ed., *Public Administration and Policy: Selected Essays* (New York: Harper & Row, 1966), pp. 58-90.

40. Anthony Downs, *Inside Bureaucracy*, A RAND Corporation Research Study (Boston: Little, Brown and Co., 1967), pp. 5ff.

41. Cf. William Robbins, "Grain Export Study Found Neglect of Safeguards," The *New York Times*, June 17, 1975, 1:6.

42. On the ups and downs of the FDA, see Miles, *The Department of Health, Education, and Welfare*, pp. 220ff.

43. Cf. Herbert C. Morton, *Public Contracts and Private Wages: Experience Under the Walsh Healy Act* (Washington: The Brookings Institution, 1965).

44. Cf. Hilton, "Basic Behavior of Regulatory Commissions," p. 48; Clark C. Havighurst, "Regulation of Health Facilities and Services by 'Certificate of Need'," 59, *Virginia Law Review* (October 1973), p. 1215.

45. Cf. Cary, *Politics and the Regulatory Agencies*, p. 79 *et. passim.*

46. Speech by Congressman John E. Moss before the Consumer Federation of America, June 11, 1975 (processed), p. 23.

47. Cf. James Q. Wilson, "The Bureaucracy Problem," VI, *The Public Interest* (Winter 1967), pp. 3-9; Jaffe, "The Illusion of Ideal Administration."

48. Cf. Noll, *Reforming Regulation*, p. 5, who draws very different implications.

49. Cf. Roger G. Noll, "The Consequences of Public Utility Regulation of Hospitals," in Institute of Medicine, National Academy of Sciences, *Controls on Health Care*, Proceedings of the Conference on Regulation in the Health Industry, January 7-9, 1974 (Washington: National Academy of Sciences, 1975), p. 33; Havighurst, "Regulation of Health Facilities," p. 1215; and, more quantitatively, George J. Stigler and Claire Friedland, "What Can Regulators Regulate?: The Case of Electricity," V, *Journal of Law and Economics* (October 1962), pp. 1-16.

50. Cf. The National Health Planning and Resources Development Act of 1974 (PL 93-641), Sec. 1533 (d) (1); also A.J.G. Priest, "Possible Adaptation of Public Utility Concepts in the Health Care Field," 35, *Law and Contemporary Problems* (Autumn 1970), p. 841.

51. Mueller and Gibson, "National Health Expenditures," p. 3.

52. Cf. Robert M. Ball, "Background of Regulation in Health Care," in Institute of Medicine, *Controls on Health Care*, pp. 11, 21; and Noll, "Consequences of Public Utility Regulation," p. 45.

53. Cf. Donald J. Dewey, "Regulatory Reform?" in William C. Shepherd and Thomas C. Gies, eds., *Regulation in Further Perspective: The Little Engine That Might* (Cambridge, Mass.: Ballinger, 1974), p. 37; Havighurst, "Regulation of Health Facilities," p. 1186; Hilton, "Basic Behavior of Regulatory Commissions," p. 50

54. Barry Ensmiger, *The $8 Billion Hospital Bed Overrun: A Consumer's Guide to Stopping Wasteful Construction*, Public Citizen's Health Research Group (Washington: Health Research Group, 1975).

55. Cf. "Editorial: Are There Too Many Hospital Beds?" 49, *Hospitals* (April 1, 1975), pp. 17-18.

56. William J. Bicknell and Diana Chapman Walsh, "Certificate of Need: The Massachusetts Experience," 292, *New England Journal of Medicine* (May 15, 1975), p. 1060.

57. Cf. Ibid., pp. 4-75.

58. Havighurst, "Regulation of Health Facilities," pp. 1207ff.

59. Cf. Cohen, "Professional Licensure."

60. Committee on Government Operations, *Program Fraud and Abuse.*

61. Cf. James M. Naughton, "President Vows He Will Reduce Industry Curbs," The *New York Times*, June 18, 1975, 1:8.

62. Cf. Adams and Adams, "The Military-Industrial Complex," pp. 279-280; Ellsworth, "Defense Procurement," p. 228.

63. Cf. Robert J. Art, *The TFX Decision: McNamara and the Military* (Boston: Little, Brown and Co., 1968), pp. 100-102.

64. See the articles by George C. Eads and Thomas Gale Moore, and the editor's introduction, in Almarin Phillips, ed., *Promoting Competition in Regulated Markets*, Studies in the Regulation of Economic Activity (Washington: The Brookings Institution, 1975); Posner, "Natural Monopoly," pp. 593ff.; Noll, *Reforming Regulation*, pp. 98-99; James W. McKie, "The Ends and Means of Regulation," General Series Reprint 287 (Washington: The Brookings Institution, 1974).

65. Cf. Eads, "Competition in the Domestic Trunk Airline Industry," in Phillips, *Promoting Competition in Regulated Markets.*

66. Harvey Averch and Leland Johnson, "The Firm Under Regulatory Constraint," 52, *American Economic Review* (December 1962), pp. 1052-1069.

67. Cf. Vladeck, "Why Non-Profits Go Broke."

68. Laurence R. Tancredi and John Woods, "The Social Control of Medical Practice: Licensure Versus Output Monitoring," *The Milbank Memorial Fund Quarterly* (January 1972), Pt. 1, pp. 99-125; Fuchs, *Who Shall Live?* pp. 75-76.

69. Ibid.

70. William C. Thomas, Jr., *Nursing Homes and Public Policy: Drift and Decision in New York State* (Ithaca, N.Y.: Cornell University Press, 1969), p. 198.

71. Cf. Herbert L. Packer, *The Limits of the Criminal Sanction*, (Stanford, Calif.: Stanford University Press, 1968), pp. 277-282.

72. Cf. Harold Hinderer, "Reimbursement: Past, Present, and Future," in Graduate Program in Hospital Administration and Center for Health Administration Studies, Graduate School of Business, University of Chicago, *Public Control and Hospital Operations*, Proceedings of the Fourteenth Annual Symposium on Hospital Affairs, May 1972 (Chicago: Graduate Program 1972).

73. Cf. chapter 8.

74. Richard A. Posner, "Taxation by Regulation," 2, *Bell Journal of Economics and Management Science* (Spring 1971), pp. 22-50; Dewey, "Regulatory Reform?" p. 35; Noll, *Reforming Regulation,* pp. 17-18.

75. Cf. Lee Loevinger, "Regulation and Competition as Alternatives," 11, *Antitrust Bulletin* (January-April 1966), p. 119; Dewey, "Regulatory Reform?" p. 35.

76. Compare Miles, *The Department of Health, Education, and Welfare,* pp. 255-263, with Marilyn G. Rose, "Federal Regulation of Services to the Poor Under the Hill–Burton Act: Realities and Pitfalls," 70, *Northwestern University Law Review* (March-April 1975), pp. 168-200.

77. A Michael Spence, "Monopoly, Quality, and Regulation," 6, *The Bell Journal of Economics* (Autumn 1975), pp. 417-429.

78. Ibid.

79. Cf. Noll, *Reforming Regulation*, p. 28.

80. Cf. R.H. Egdahl and Cynthia H. Taft, "On Measuring 'Quality' Health Care: Beyond the Hospital," 294, *New England Journal of Medicine* (January 15, 1976), pp. 161-162.

81. Cf. William M. Capron, "Introduction," to Capron, ed., *Technological Change in Regulated Industries*, Studies in the Regulation of Economic Activity (Washington: The Brookings Institution, 1971), pp. 10-12.

82. Noll, "Consequences of Public Utility Regulation," pp. 35-38; Havighurst, "Regulation of Health Facilities," p. 1148; Howard Berman, "Regulation: The Public Policy Dilemma," 19, *Hospital Administration* (Fall 1974), pp. 15-16.

83. Cf. Remarks by Senator Javits, *Congressional Record*, January 27, 1976, pp. 587-589; Russell and Burke, "Technological Diffusion in the Hospital Sector;" Fuchs, *Who Shall Live?* chapter 2.

84. Noll, "Consequences of Public Utility Regulation," p. 39.

85. Cf. Packer, *Limits of the Criminal Sanction*, pp. 282ff.

86. Richard M. Titmuss, *The Gift Relationship: From Human Blood to Social Policy* (New York: Vintage Books, 1971), pp. 195ff.

87. Cf. Bernstein, *Regulating Business by Independent Commission*, pp. 179ff; Cary, *Politics and the Regulatory Agencies*, pp. 130, 132.

88. Cf. Noll, "Consequences of Public Utility Regulation," pp. 43-45.

89. Cf. Barbara and John Ehrenreich, "Health Care and Social Control," 5, *Social Policy* (May-June 1974), pp. 31-35.

90. Remarks by Mrs. Lillian Roberts, associate director, District Council 37, American Federation of State, County, and Municipal Employees, AFL-CIO, Open-House Seminar, Center for Community Health Systems, Columbia University, May 28, 1975.

91. Cf. Yeheskel Dror, "Government Decision-Making: Muddling Through, Science or Inertia," XXIV, *Public Administration Review* (September 1964), pp. 154-157.

92. Cf. American Hospital Association, "Report of the Advisory Panel on Public Utility Regulation, " April 27, 1971.

Chapter 7
The Political Economy of National Health Insurance:
Policy Analysis and Political Evaluation

1. *Washington Post*, April 3, 1976, p. A3.

2. "The Social Security Revolution," *Congressional Quarterly: Congress and the Nation*, Vol. 1 (Washington, D.C.: Congressional Quarterly Service, 1965), p. 1225.

3. T.R. Marmor, *The Politics of Medicare*, (Chicago: Aldine, 1973), p. 111.

4. Murray Edelman, *The Symbolic Uses of Politics* (Chicago: University of Illinois Press, 1964), pp. 29, 125, 134-138, 160-161.

5. Richard Nixon, "The Nation's Health Care System," *Weekly Compilation of Presidential Documents,* Vol. 5, No. 28, July 10, 1969, p. 963.

6. "Our Ailing Medical System," *Fortune*, Vol. 81, No. 1, January, 1970.

7. George Meany statement of the AFL-CIO, *Hearings on National Health Insurance*, Committee on Ways and Means, October-November 1971, p. 239.

8. Stephen P. Strickland, *U.S. Health Care: What's Right and What's Wrong* (New York: Universe Books, 1972), pp. 43, 102.

9. Council on Wage and Price Stability, "The Problem of Rising Health Care Costs," No. 81 (Washington, D.C.: The Bureau of National Affairs, Inc., April 26, 1976), p. x-4.

10. Ibid.

11. U.S., Executive Office of the President, *Budget of the United States Government 1976: Special Analysis* (Washington, D.C.: U.S. Government Printing Office, 1975), p. 170; U.S. Congress, House of Representatives, Committee on Ways and Means, *Basic Charts on Health Care* (Washington, D.C.: U.S. Government Printing Office, July 8, 1975), pp. 44-45.

12. *Budget of the United States Government 1976: Special Analysis,* pp. 183-184.

13. *Medical World News*, February 23, 1976, p. 25.

14. Brian Abel-Smith, "Value for Money in Health," *Social Security Bulletin*, Vol. 37, No. 7, July 1974, p. 18.

15. Barbara Ehrenrich and John Ehrenrich, *The American Health Empire: Power, Profit and Politics* (New York: Random House, 1970).

16. See, for example, Rick Carlson, *The End of Medicine* (New York: John Wiley & Sons, 1975).

17. See Michael Meyer, *Journal of Health Politics, Policy and Law,* Vol. 1, No. 1.

18. Martin Feldstein, "A New Approach to National Health Insurance," *The Public Interest,* 1971. This is only one version of Feldstein's MRI. See discussion later in the chapter.

19. Saul Waldman, *National Health Insurance Proposals: Provisions of Bills Introduced in the 93rd Congress of July 1974,* DHEW Publications No. (SSA) 75-11920, pp. 194-195.

20. S.3; HR23, 1975.

21. Waldman, *National Health Insurance Proposals,* pp. 16, 161; John Holahan, *Financing Health Care for the Poor* (Boston: D.C. Heath and Co., 1975), pp. 86-90.

22. AMA Statement on National Health Insurance (by Dr. Max Parrot), *Hearings on National Health Insurance,* Ways and Means Committee, October-November 1971, p. 1951.

23. Ibid.

24. Feldstein, "A New Approach to National Health Insurance"; "National Health Insurance: Which Way to Go?" *Consumer Reports,* February 1975.

25. Rashi Fein, *The Doctor Shortage* (Washington: The Brookings Institution, 1967), Chapter 1.

26. D. Lynch, National Health Council, *Declaration of Independence,* p. 35.

27. See, among others, comments by Michael Zubkoff in The National Health Council, *Declaration of Independence,* p. 62.

28. See U.S. Congress, House, Committee on Ways and Means, *National Health Insurance, Panel Discussion,* before the Subcommittee on Health July 10, 11, 17, 24, and September 12, 1975, 94th Congress, 1st Session (Washington, D.C.: U.S. Government Printing Office, 1975).

29. Rashi Fein, *The Doctor Shortage*; Martin Feldstein, "The Rising Price of Physicians' Services," *Review of Economics and Statistics,* May 1970.

30. See "Health Insurance: No Action in 1974," *Congressional Quarterly, Almanac: 93rd Congress 2nd Session,* (Washington, D.C.: Congressional Quarterly Service, 1965), pp. 386-394. John K. Iglehart, "Health Report/Mills Switch Fails to Bring Approval for Insurance Plan," *National Journal Reports,* August 24, 1974, pp. 1267-1268.

31. See John K. Iglehart, "Health Report/Jobless Medical Aid Debate Forcuses on Financing Method," *National Journal Reports,* March 29, 1975, pp. 457-463; Iglehart, "Health Report/Feuding, Ford Opposition Perils Jobless Health Insurance," *National Journal Reports,* April 19, 1975, pp. 592-594; Iglehart, "Health Report/Speaker Supports Rogers in Dispute With Ways and

Means," *National Journal Reports*, May 24, 1975, p. 773; *Congressional Quarterly Weekly Report* (Washington, D.C., Congressional Quarterly Service, 1975), pp. 537-540, 608-609, 769-770, 809-810, 879-880, 927-928, 1034, 1091-1095.

32. Iglehart, "Jobless Medical Aid Debate Focuses on Financing Method," p. 458.

33. Ibid., pp. 462-463.

34. Marmor, *The Politics of Medicare*, pp. 59-60.

35. See John F. Manley, *The Politics of Finance: The House Committee on Ways and Means* (Boston: Little, Brown, 1970); Richard F. Fenno, Jr., *Congressmen in Committees* (Boston: Little, Brown, 1973); Kenneth M. Bowler, *The Nixon Guaranteed Income Proposal*, (Cambridge: Balinger, 1974), pp. 83-123.

36. See Theodore R. Marmor, *The Politics of Medicare;* (Chicago: Aldine, 1973), James L. Sundquist, *Politics and Policy,* (Washington, D.C.: Brookings Institution, 1968); and Bowler, *Nixon Guaranteed Income Proposal,* pp. 123-173.

Chapter 8
The Medical Care System Under National Health Insurance:
Four Models

1. M. Feldstein and B. Friedman, "Tax Subsidies, the Rational Demand for Insurance and the Health Care Crisis," Discussion Paper No. 382, Harvard Institute of Economic Research, Sept. 1974.

2. R. Rosett and L. Huang, "The Effect of Health Insurance on the Demand for Medical Care," *Journal of Political Economy* 81 (March 1973): 281 and M. Feldstein, "The Welfare Loss of Excess Health Insurance," *J. Pol. Econ.* 81 (March 1973): 251.

3. M. Mueller, "Private Health Insurance in 1973," *Social Security Bulletin* (Feb. 1975): 21.

4. *Report of the Catastrophic Illness Conference* (Rockville, Md.: National Center for Health Services Research, HEW, Dec. 1, 1974).

5. N. Kouchoukos et al., "An Appraisal of Coronary Bypass Grafting," *Circulation* 50 (July 1974): 11 and E. Corday, "Status of Coronary Bypass Surgery," *Journal of the American Medical Association* 231 (Mar. 24, 1975): 1245.

6. H. Hiatt, "Protecting the Medical Commons," *New England Journal of Medicine* 293 (July 31, 1975): 235.

7. Center for Health Policy Research, *Health Insurance: What Should Be the Federal Role?* (Washington: American Enterprise Institute, Jan. 22, 1975).

8. R. Anderson, Testimony in Hearings on National Health Insurance before the Subcommittee on Public Health and Environment of the House Committee on Interstate and Foreign Commerce, 93rd U.S. Congress, Dec. 14, 1973.

9. K. Davis, "Health Insurance," in C. Schultze, et al., *Setting National Priorities: the 1973 Budget* (Washington: Brookings Institution, 1973), p. 213.

10. L. Aday and R. Anderson, *Access to Medical Care* (Ann Arbor, Michigan: Health Administration Press, 1975) and D. Kessner, "Myths Revisited: National Health Insurance Improves the Health of the Poor," 102nd Annual Meeting of A.P.H.A. Oct. 22, 1974. See also R. Wilson and E. White, "Changes in Morbidity, Disability and Utilization . . . 1964 and 1973," ibid.

11. "Utilization of Short-Stay Hospitals in 1971," National Health Survey Series 13, No. 7, HEW, 1974. See also, "Surgical Operations in Short-Stay Hospitals," Series 13, No. 18, ibid and J. Wennberg and A. Gittelsohn, "Small Area Variations in Health Care Delivery," *Science* 182 (Dec. 14, 1973): 1102.

12. R. Maxwell, *Health Care, the Growing Dilemma* (N.Y.: McKinsey & Co., 1974).

13. R. Auster et al.,"The Production of Health," *Journal of Human Resources* 4 (Fall 1969): 411. See also, for example: N. Glazer, "Paradoxes of Health Care," *Public Interest* 22 (Winter 1971): 62; W. Barton,"Infant Mortality and Health Insurance Coverage," *Inquiry* 9 (Sept. 1972): 16; and "Regional Variations in Mortality from Heart Disease," *Statistical Bulletin of the Metropolitan Life Insurance Co.* (Nov. 1972): 3.

14. P. Ellwood, et al., *Assuring the Quality of Health Care* (Minneapolis, Minn.: InterStudy, 1973), Chap 3 and R. Brook, "Critical Issues in the Assessment of Quality of Care," *Journal of Medical Education* 48, Part 2 (April 1973): 114.

15. M. Mueller and R. Gibson, "National Health Expenditures," *Social Security Bulletin* (Feb. 1976).

16. C. Schultze et al., *Setting National Priorities, the 1973 Budget.*

17. B. Stuart and R. Stockton, "Control over the Utilization of Medical Services," *Milbank Memorial Fund Quarterly* 51 (Summer 1973): 341. See also *Rising Medical Costs in Michigan* (Report of the Technical Work Group on Health Care Costs, Michigan Dept. of Social Services, Lansing, July 1973) and P. O'Donoghue et al., *An Evaluation of Policy Related Research on the Effects of Health Care Regulation* (Denver: Policy Center, Inc., 1975).

18. Several terms are used in the analysis which are defined here. By "effectiveness" is meant the degree of improved health levels in the population cared for, within the limits that health care can improve health. "Quality" of health care is defined synonymously with effectiveness. By "efficiency" is meant effectiveness divided by cost; i.e., we understand efficiency as health improvement per dollar expended, not number of services per dollar expended.

By "style" of practice is meant the degree of use of costly, technological inputs. "High style" means a high level of costly inputs; high style health care can be effective or ineffective, but it is always high cost. "Low style" practice makes less use of costly inputs; it can be effective or ineffective, just as with high style care, but it always costs less per service. Of course, ineffective low style care could eventually cost more than effective high style care. Conversely, equally effective low style care is more efficient than high style care.

19. J. Bunker and B. Brown, "The Physician Patient as an Informed Consumer of Surgical Services," *New England Journal of Medicine* 290 (May 9, 1974): 1051.

20. J. McLamb and R. Huntley, "Hazards of Hospitalization," *Southern Medical Journal* 60 (1967): 469–72. See also E. Schimmel, "Hazards of Hospitalization," *Annual of Internal Medicine* 60 (1964): 100–110; and note 32.

21. C. Aring, "The Place of the Physician in Modern Society," *Journal of the American Medical Association* 228 (Apr. 8, 1974): 177.

22. *Profile of Medical Practice in 1974* (Chicago: American Medical Association, 1974) Tables 50, 52 64. See also note 51.

23. J. Maloney, "A Report on the Role of Economic Motivation in the Performance of Medical School Faculty," *Surgery* 68 (July 1970): 1. See also, M. Roemer, "On Paying the Doctor and the Implications of Different Methods," *Journal of Health and Human Behavior* 3 (Spring 1962): 4.

24. J. Simanis, "International Health Expenditures," *Social Security Bulletin* (Dec. 1970): 18. See also notes 12 and 68.

25. See note 3.

26. C. Havighurst, "Statement . . . on HMO's," Testimony in Hearings before the Senate Subcommittee on Monopoly and Antitrust, U.S. Congress (May 15, 1974). See also R. Trussel, et al., *The Quantity, Quality and Costs of Medical and Hospital Care Secured by a Sample of Teamster Families in New York City* (New York: School of Public Health, Columbia University, 1972).

27. M. Bennett, "Health Insurance, Medical Need and Hospital Consumption," *Inquiry* 12 (March, 1975): 59–66.

28. See note 14.

29. M. Feldstein, "Hospital Cost Inflation," *American Economic Review* 61 (Dec. 1971): 853. See also K. Davis, "An Empirical Investigation of Alternative Models of the Hospital Industry," Annual Meeting of American Economic Association, Toronto, Dec. 30, 1972.

30. A. Donabedian, "An Evaluation of Prepaid Group Practice," *Inquiry* 6 (Sept. 1969): 3; M. Roemer and W. Shonick, "HMO Performance," *Milbank Memorial Fund Quarterly* 51, (Summer 1973): 271 and M. Corbin and A. Krute, "Some Aspects of Medicare Experience with Group Practice Prepayment Plans," *Social Security Bulletin* (March 1973): 3.

31. See notes 14, 30 and C. Snow, "Do the Poor Receive Poor Quality Medical Care?" 102nd Annual Meeting of American Public Health Association, New Orleans, Oct. 24, 1972.

32. C. Lewis, "Variations in the Incidence of Surgery," *New England Journal of Medicine* 281 (Oct. 16, 1969): 880. See also E. Vayda, "A Comparison of Surgical Rates in Canada and in England and Wales," *New England Journal of Medicine* 289 (Dec. 6 1973): 1224 and J. Bunker and J. Wennberg, ibid, 1249.

33. See note 11.

34. Ibid.

35. See notes 13, 34, and A. Cochrane, *Effectiveness and Efficiency* (England: Nuffield Provincial Hospitals Trust, 1971).

36. See notes 6, 14, 27, 34, and D. Spodick, "Numerators without Denominators," *Journal of American Medical Association* 232 (April 7, 1975): 35.

37. F. Sattler and M. Bennett, *A Statistical Profile of Short Term Hospitals in the United States in 1973* (Minneapolis: InterStudy, 1975); B. Ensminger, *The $8 Billion Hospital Bed Overrun* (Washington: Public Citizen's Health Research Group, 1975) and Report to the Congress by the Comptroller General, *Study of Health Facilities Construction Costs* (Washington: U.S. Government Printing Office, 1972).

38. Report to the Congress.

39. E. Brian, *Government Control of Hospital Utilization* (Sacramento, California: Dept. of Health Services, 1971).

40. E. McCarthy and G. Widmer, "Effects of Screening by Consultants on Recommended Surgical Procedures," *New England Journal of Medicine* 291 (Dec. 19, 1974): 1331.

41. S. Bellin et al., "Impact of Ambulatory Health Care Services on the Demand for Hospital Beds," *New England Journal of Medicine* 15 (April 10, 1969): 808.

42. P. Gertman and B. Bucher, "Inappropriate Bed Days and the Relationship to Length of Stay Parameters," Paper presented at the 99th Meeting of the American Public Health Association, Minneapolis, Oct. 11, 1971.

43. See note 17.

44. T. Kelly and G. Schieber, *Factors Affecting Medical Services Utilization* (Washington: Urban Institute, Dec. 1972).

45. D. Harris, "An Elaboration of the Relationship Between General Hospital Bed Supply and General Hospital Utilization," *Journal of Social Behavior* 15 (June 1975): 163. See also note 51.

46. R. Stevens, "Trends in Medical Specialization," *Inquiry* 8 (Mar. 1971): 9.

47. J. Chamberlain, "Selected Data on Group Practice Prepayment Plan Services," *Group Health and Welfare News*, Special Supplement, June 1967.

48. Although the cost and distribution problems (Section II) are mainly due to the insulation of specialists from market pressures, perhaps the largest voice in the AMA is the general and family practitioners, who live in a rather more competitive environment. This may play some role in the AMA's failure to perceive the real problems or to come up with a credible strategy for the medical care system.

49. *Distribution of Physicians and Hospitals* (Chicago: American Medical Association, 1970). However, see also, J. Sparks, "Physician Maldistribution?" *Private Practice* (Sept. 1972).

50. "Availability and Use of Health Services," *Agricultural Economic Report No. 139* (Washington: U.S. Dept. of Agriculture, July 1968).

51. V. Fuchs and M. Kramer, *Determinants of Expenditures for Physicians Services* (Rockville, Md.: National Center for Health Services Research, Dec. 1972).

52. J. Kasper et al., *The Financial Impact of Catastrophic Illness as Measured in the CHAS-NORC National Survey* (Chicago: Center for Health Admin. Studies, Univ. of Chicago, 1975).

53. The NHI proposals of the American Medical Association suggest that they missed this lesson. Because they expand financing with no credible strategy to contain costs, these proposals are the most likely to hasten the draconian regulation they fear.

54. We stress how powerful these incentives are. For example, given existing excess hospital capacity in the nation, if these controls were to work they would force many hospitals into financial jeopardy if not outright bankruptcy (see note 37). Again, the amount of specialty work would have to decline substantially. Hospitals and specialists both will work to circumvent the controls.

55. The evidence suggests that good clinicians may ignore up to half or more of the procedural steps usually included in explicit procedure-based standards. In other words, they use experience and judgment to adjust the procedural mix to the individual patient in ways impossible to formulate into a standard, which must include every step that might be relevant. See R. Brook, "Quality of Care Assessment, Policy Relevant Issues," *Policy Sciences* 5 (Sept. 1974): 317. Outcome studies support their skill in this. Poor end results seem far more often the result of idiosyncratic system linkage failures (between provider and patient, provider and provider, provider and appointment desk, etc.) which seldom appear in standards, and only infrequently are due to omitted or poorly done medical procedures (see note 14). On the other hand, if cost control begins to pinch, it can easily be imagined that providers will follow all procedural standards to the letter, and there will be no objective way to fault them medically. Cost will be forced up with no improvement in health.

56. R. Brook, "Quality of Care Assessment, Policy Relevant Issues."

57. R. Noll, *Reforming Regulation* (Brookings Institution, Washington, D.C.,

1971). See also, W. Jordan, "Procedure Protection, Prior Market Structure, and the Effects of Government Regulation," *Journal of Law and Economics* 15 (1972): 151.

58. See note 17.

59. "Monthly Statistical Report: Summary of Selected Price, Costs, and Utilization Data for the Health Care Market in the United States," Social Security Administration Office of Research and Statistics, Dec. 1972.

60. See note 15.

61. M. Feldstein, "A New Approach to National Health Insurance," *Public Interest (Spring 1971) and M. Pauly, National Health Insurance: An Analysis* (Washington: American Enterprise Institute, 1971).

62. C. Phelps and J. Newhouse, *Coinsurance and the Demand for Medical Services* (Santa Monica, Cal.: Rand, Report R-964-1-OEO, Oct. 1974).

63. There are no research studies comparing health outcomes in matched populations with and without heavy income-related cost-sharing, and further research is needed. The studies looking at service use under non-income-related copayments did not look at health outcomes, but the service variations found did not seem a priori threatening to health. See A. Scitovsky and N. Snyder, "Effect of Coinsurance on the Use of Physicians Services," *Social Security Bulletin* (June 1972): 3 and R. Beck, "An Analysis of the Demand for Physician Services in Saskatchewan," Ph.D. Thesis, University of Alberta, Edmonton, Spring 1971. Some preventive services were foregone by some persons, but society could subsidize such services if wished.

64. Although data on catastrophic benefits are sketchy, it appears that a substantial number of the population presently have inadequate or no catastrophic protection. One piece of evidence is the number of persons without major medical or comprehensive benefits, roughly estimated at somewhere less than half the population. See M. Mueller, "Private Health Insurance in 1970," *Social Security Bulletin* (Feb. 1972): 3; *Sourcebook of Health Insurance,* 1973–74 (N.Y.: Health Insurance Institute, 1974); and *A Current Profile of Group Medical Expense Insurance in Force in the U.S.* (N.Y.: Health Insurance Association of America, Feb. 1974). The other evidence is that persons incurring large medical expenditures have unrepresentatively high incomes relative to the U.S. average (see R. Anderson), implying that lower income persons are inhibited by lack of coverage or stiff cost-sharing at the catastrophic end. (See F. Sloan and B. Steinwald. "Role of Health Insurance," *Inquiry* 12 [Dec. 1974] : 275.) This disagrees with the conclusion of J. Newhouse et al. (see J. Newhouse et al., "Policy Options and the Impact of National Health Insurance," *New England Journal of Medicine* 290 [June 13, 1974] : 1345), that catastrophic care is well covered presently. But Newhouse et al. do agree that technology could make catastrophic care very inflationary.

65. See note 4 and W. McClure, Testimony in Hearings on National Health Insurance before the House Committee on Ways and Means, 93rd U.S. Congress, May 10, 1974.

66. "A New Approach."

67. M. Mueller, "Private Health Insurance in 1970."

68. R. Eilers (dec.), Leonard Davis, Inst. Health Economics, University of Pennsylvania, personal communication.

69. R. Evans, "Health Care Costs and Expenditures in Canada," Proceedings of the International Conference on Health Costs and Expenditures, Fogarty International Center, National Institute of Health, Washington, D.C., 1975, (to be published); also in *National Health Insurance: Can We Learn From Canada?*, ed: S. Andreopolos, (John Wiley, New York, 1975). Saskatchewan instituted modest copayments in their previously full coverage plan in 1969, which were discontinued after a couple of years. California instituted copayments in Medicaid in 1973, which have been discontinued presently.

70. P. Ellwood, et al., "The Health Maintenance Strategy," *Medical Care* 9 (May 1971): 291.

71. See note 65.

72. Brook, "Critical Issues," Donabedian, "An Evaluation," and C. Snow, "Do the Poor Receive Poor Quality Medical Care?"

73. J. Iglehart, "HMO Act Changes Advanced to Bolster Troubled Program," *National Journal Reports* (August 16, 1975): 1161.

74. For a more skeptical view, see U. Reinhardt, "Proposed Changes in the Organization of Health-Care Delivery: An Overview and Critique," *Milbank Memorial Fund Quarterly* (Spring 1973): 196-222.

75. See note 72.

76. "A Review of the Regulation of Prepaid Health Plans by the State Department of Health," Legislative Analyst Report, State Capitol, Sacramento, Cal., Nov. 15, 1973.

77. See note 32.

78. See Ellwood, et al., "Assuring the Quality" and Brooks, "Quality of Care Assessment."

79. Ellwood, et al., "Health Maintenance Strategy" and McClure, "Testimony."

80. Iglehart, "HMO Act."

81. R. Noll, "Public Utility Regulation of Hospitals," mimeograph, Dept. of Econ., Cal. Inst. of Technology, Oct. 3, 1973. See also C. Havighurst, "Certificate of Need Laws and Franchising Proposals," mimeograph, School of Law, Duke University, Oct. 31, 1972; and note 57.

82. G. Silver, "Fair Shares, the U.S.A. is Ready for a National Health Service," *Pharos* (July 1973): 95.

83. Maxwell, "Health Care."

84. Simanis, "International Health Expenditures."

85. W. Flash, *Political Implications of National Health Insurance Proposals* (Indiana Public Health Foundation, Fall 1970), p. 13.

86. See note 69.

87. Mueller and Gibson, "National Health Expenditures."

88. O'Donoghue, et al., "An Evaluation;" Stuart and Stocton, "Control;" and F. Sattler, *Hospital Prospective Rate Setting* (Minneapolis: InterStudy, Mar. 1975)

89. A. Somers, *Health Care in Transition* (Chicago: The Hospital Research and Educational Trust, 1971).

90. R. Schulz and J. Rose, "Can Hospitals Be Expected to Contain Costs?" *Inquiry* 10 (June 1973): 3.

91. C. Lewis and H. Kairnes, "Controlling Costs of Medical Care by Expanding Insurance Coverage," *New England Journal of Medicine* 282 (June 18, 1970): 1405.

92. "Hospital Guide Issue," *Hospitals: Journal of the American Hospital Association* (Aug. 1974).

93. See note 81.

94. This should spur a new interest in shared services but for very different motives: by government helping to encourage efficiency, and by hospitals hoping to initiate alliances.

95. U. Reinhardt, "Proposed Changes."

96. G. Clarke, "Health Programs in the States," (Eagleton Inst. of Politics, Rutgers University, Mar. 1975).

97. M. Doody, "Status of Multi-Hospital Systems," *Hospitals* 48 (June 1, 1974): 61. See also M. Brown, "Current Trends in Cooperative Ventures," ibid.

98. For an opposite view, see H. Klarman, "Major Public Initiatives in Health Care," *Public Interest* 34 (Winter 1974): 106-23.

99. D. Greenberg, "Preparing for National Health Insurance and Other Matters," *New England Journal of Medicine* 291 (Nov. 28, 1974): 1205.

100. The stringency of incentive reimbursement should not be tied to superficial efficiency criteria such as occupancy; clearly, if the HSAs are successful at reducing hospital days per capita, existing hospitals will be running at lower occupancy unless we close beds. Reimbursement formulae might better become more stringent based on keeping average hospital days per capita in the area, and average hospital days per staff physician in each hospital, within desired tolerances.

101. The AMA, for example, spent great effort fighting the HMO Act, which is an effort to reform and maintain a pluralistic, private system of medicine, whereas they gave rather token opposition to PSRO (perhaps because they believe doctors will run it), which creates an administrative structure with powerful regulatory potential where nothing existed before.

About the Contributors

Kenneth M. Bowler received the B.A. from Stanford University and the Ph.D. from the University of Wisconsin, Madison. He served as an American Political Science Association Congressional Fellow in 1970 and 1971. From 1971 to 1974 he was on the faculty of the Political Science Department of the University of Maryland–Baltimore County, and is presently on the staff of the Committee of Ways and Means of the U.S. House of Representatives. He is author of *The Nixon Guaranteed Income Proposal: Substance and Process in Policy Change* (Ballinger, 1974).

Judith M. Feder is nearing completion of the Ph.D. in government at Harvard University. Her essay in this volume is the result of a long-term study begun while she held a fellowship at the Brookings Institution, and continued under contract from the Social Security Administration to Spectrum Research, Inc. She is presently a service fellow at the National Center for Health Services Research.

Thomas R. Fulda, social science research analyst on the staff of the Drug Studies Branch, Office of Research and Statistics, Social Security Administration, obtained the B.A. from Lawrence University, Appleton, Wisconsin in political science and the M.A. from the University of Michigan. His major research has been in the field of expenditures for prescription drugs under federal, state, and local government reimbursement programs. He has also done research on comparative efforts to control the cost of prescription drugs.

Robert T. Kudrle is assistant professor of public affairs at the University of Minnesota and has served as assistant director and acting director of the University's Harold Scott Quigley Center of International Studies. He received the Ph.D. in economics from Harvard University where he was a graduate research associate at the Center for International Affairs. He also holds the B.Phil. in economics from Oxford University and the A.B. in government from Harvard. Dr. Kudrle is the author of *Agricultural Tractors: A World Industry Study* (Ballinger, 1975) and several articles on industrial organization, international political economy, and public policy.

T.R. Marmor is associate professor in the School of Social Service Administration and in the College of the University of Chicago, and research associate of the Center for Health Administration Studies there. He is author of *The Politics of Medicare* (Aldine, 1973) and *Poverty Policy* (Aldine-Atherton, 1973), as well as a frequent contributor to the journals in social policy and politics, and a consultant to federal and state agencies. He is now completing a book on the implementation problems of national health insurance.

Walter McClure is senior policy analyst and director of the Health Policy Group, at InterStudy, a private independent nonprofit organization located in Minneapolis, which is devoted to improving health-care delivery and financing. His principal interests have been in organized delivery systems, evaluation of medical care by patient outcomes and national health insurance. He has been consultant to Congress and the administration on policies pertaining to the above fields.

Jane Cassels Record, senior economist, Kaiser Foundation Health Services Research Center, has published several monographs and nearly 100 articles in journals ranging from *The American Economic Review* to *The New Yorker*. Recently she has concentrated on health manpower research and on completing a Guggenheim study of the rural south.

Richard A. Rettig is a political scientist in the Washington office of the Rand Corporation. His research concerns health and federal research and development policy. A book, *Cancer Crusade: The Story of the National Cancer Act of 1971* will be published by the Princeton University Press in 1977.

Bruce C. Vladeck received the Ph.D. in political science from The University of Michigan. After being on the staff of the New York City-Rand Institute, he assumed his present position as assistant professor of public health (health administration) and political science in the Center for Community Health Systems at Columbia University. He has written widely on health policy and general public policy.

Thomas C. Webster is assistant professor of public administration at the Institute of Public Administration at The Pennsylvania State University. He received the Ph.D. from Ohio State University. His current research centers on public-sector productivity and on health financing and delivery systems.

About the Editors

Kenneth M. Friedman is assistant professor of political science at Purdue University. He received the B.A. from Queens College, City University of New York, and the M.A. and Ph.D. from Michigan State University. He is the author of *Public Policy and the Smoking Health Controversy: A Comparative Study* (D.C. Heath and Co., 1975) and has a continuing interest in the comparative analysis of health-care politics and policy. He teaches courses relating to science, technology, and public policy and spent the past summer as a consultant to the National Research Council's Committee on Nuclear and Alternative Energy Systems, examining transportation conservation-demand alternatives for the 1976-2010 time period.

Stuart H. Rakoff is assistant director of Research and Statistics for the United Mine Workers of America Health and Retirement Funds. He holds the Ph.D. in political science from the University of Minnesota and has previously published articles in the area of public policy analysis, especially of local governments, and in computer-assisted instructional materials. His present research centers on the operation and impact of third-party payers in the health-care system.